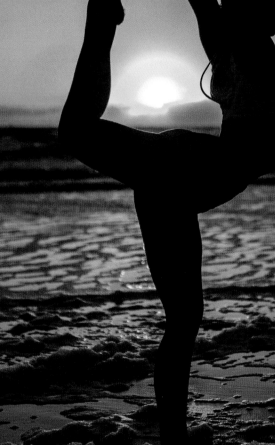

SHINE
ON & OFF
THE MAT

VERONIQUE ORY

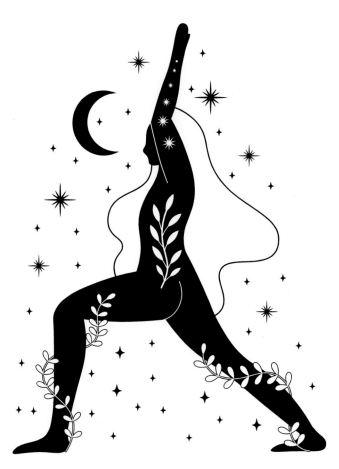

Join me in this exploration over a year of unique timely and timeless themes, stories, featured poses, dynamic sequences, curated playlists, inspirational quotes, and corresponding journal prompts. Each entry will be accompanied by a photo, which represents the theme and energy of each practice. Turn up the music and practice along with me in my on-demand series on my Vimeo channel. Read, move, find stillness and carry the yoga teachings with you in all you do.

<u>My Spotify</u>

<u>My Vimeo Channel</u>

Shine On & Off the Mat

Veronique Ory

ISBN (Print Edition): 978-1-66782-491-8

ISBN (eBook Edition): 978-1-66782-492-5

Dedicated to my students.
You teach me more than you know.

"Here's to the crazy ones. The misfits. The rebels. The troublemakers. The round pegs in the square holes. The ones who see things differently. They're not fond of rules. And they have no respect for the status quo. You can quote them, disagree with them, glorify or vilify them. About the only thing you can't do is ignore them. Because they change things. They push the human race forward. And while some may see them as the crazy ones, we see genius. Because the people who are crazy enough to think they can change the world, are the ones who do."

– Rob Siltanen

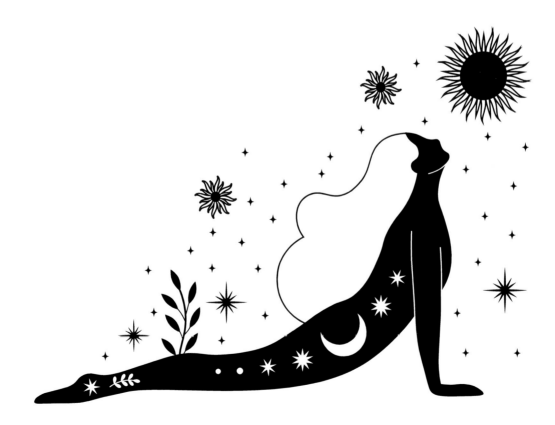

The ideal guide for those desiring long term structure and gentle guidance for their movement and creative practices. Veronique brings her signature organization and logical, but creative and unique style to this inclusive and accessible offering. Whether you're wanting asana, introspective journaling, exquisite storytelling and theme work, or all of the above, you'll find it in *Shine On & Off the Mat*. You don't want to miss this!

STEPH GÓNGORA

E-RYT 500

Veronique's innovative book empowers a holistic yoga experience by combining the physical, mental and spiritual aspects of yoga. Her comprehensive teaching style is sure to deepen your practice, and her artistic touch with music and with words is an inspiration to experience.

DANA SLAMP

C-IAYT, FOUNDER, PREMA YOGA INSTITUTE

My favorite yoga teacher pours her heart and soul into the most perfect guide for anyone looking to discover themselves through the journey of yoga. Follow along to peel back all the layers of the self as Veronique so passionately and eloquently gives readers journal prompts, themes and shapes to follow. Full of captivating photos, inspiration and beauty. A must read for any level yogi.

ASHLY BILLE

FOUNDER AND DIRECTOR OF
RHYTHM & SOUL IN VERO BEACH, FL

Shine On & Off The Mat is a warm invitation to take a beautifully curated journey through the practice of yoga on and off the mat. Veronique shares her authentic warmth and love for the practice so beautifully. Reading these pages you will feel like someone is holding sacred space for you, and that's because in her words and in curation Veronique literally is holding space for every reader. Perfect for anyone ready to dive into a deeper journey into the self through Yoga.

JUSTIN RANDOLPH

YOGA TEACHER, REIKI MASTER, + DIRECTOR
OF YOGA LOFT MANHATTAN BEACH

When a teacher opens their heart and offers insight into the inner process of engineered and designed teachings, it is a golden opportunity for us to reflect on the full spectrum of what is being shared with us as students. Through her new book, Veronique allows us to share in her inner approach to the yoga practice and her style of teaching yoga. It is a real inspiration when teachers are this open and giving. We should all take note of that openness.

AUSTIN SANDERSON

FOUNDER OF THE URBAN SADHU YOGA METHOD
AND CO-FOUNDER OF URBAN SADHU BEAUTY

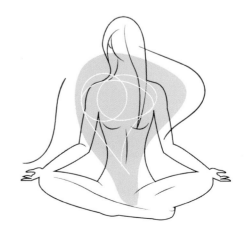

Shine On & Off The Mat is such a treasure! In its multidimensional formatting, Veronique has created a resource of exceptional depth and tremendous accessibility that serves both new + seasoned yogis alike. This playful and dynamic book is a must-have for anyone looking to expand their awareness and connection to self, others, and the Universe at large.

EMILY CASSEL

SOULFUL BUSINESS + LEADERSHIP COACH
FOR WOMEN ENTREPRENEURS, HOST OF
LIKE NOBODY'S BUSINESS PODCAST, + AUTHOR

Veronique has mastered the dance of challenging while nurturing, of pushing and then letting go. Her teaching is marked by endless innovation, confidence in her students' abilities, and a deep sense of the end game: feeling like your best self. This book is the perfect expression of her world. You will be lucky to enter it.

SUSANNA AARON

ADORING STUDENT

I couldn't love this offering more. More than a book, it is an experience and proposes a way in which you can not only work on your yoga practice, but link it very directly to your daily life. This gives you a way to digest and try on the information through a wonderful mix of reading and writing. Truly a beautiful expression of how story can meet practice to heal the heart and body.

MILES BORRERO

YOGA TEACHER

Veronique Ory's *Shine On & Off the Mat* led me through a transformational journey along side her own. Embodied in her themed practices, storytelling, music, quotes, and journal prompts is her quest to confront everyday challenges for herself and the reader; allowing each to be both student and teacher. Through her exploration I found the motivation and inspiration to delve into myself, to be humble and receptive to change and growth, both on and off the mat, with gratitude. This exploration, and in turn, strength, has become a part of my every day now. I am so thankful for the complete and comprehensive mind body journey Veronique led me through with this incredible compilation.

KARYN PAPPAS

FASHION STYLIST, NYC

This is so much more than your typical Yoga book. It's a guided practice on cultivating mindsets necessary for staying calm, reflective, and eager to learn; using movement as the driver on this path. Highly recommend!

ZAC CUPPLES

PHYSICAL THERAPIST. ZACCUPPLES.COM

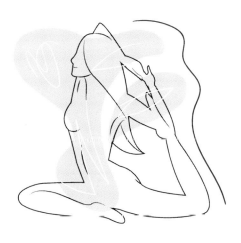

THEMES FOR
SHINE ON & OFF THE MAT

EPILOGUE PRACTICES

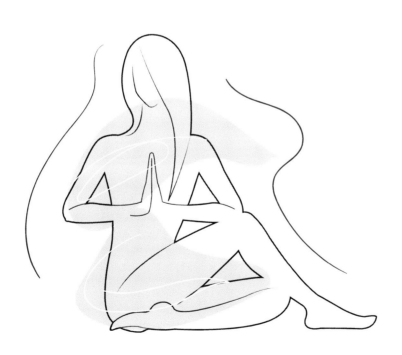

 Veronique Ory's Videos

 Veronique Ory's Playlists

INTRODUCTION

Hello, and welcome to my yoga book! I'm grateful that you've picked it up. My name is Veronique Ory. I'm an RYT (Registered Yoga Teacher with Yoga Alliance) 500 yoga instructor with a passion for weaving storytelling and unique sequences into each of my classes, inviting my students to carry their yoga practice with them on and off the mat.

This book and my practices are for the enthusiastic yogi, whether you are beginning your yoga journey or a long-time practitioner. I invite you to read, practice, and listen with an open heart. My offerings are tailored to curious souls seeking transformation through timely and timeless themes.

The inspiration to write this book came from Brandon, who encouraged me to write down the dharma talks I regularly give to my classes. I began doing so seven weeks before the pandemic, thinking that what I ended up with would be more of a memoir or personal journal of sorts. When the pandemic hit and I created my own Vimeo channel, I began to think it could be a yearlong catalogue. I had never seen an interactive yoga book of this kind, which syncs up storytelling with playlists, on-demand classes, journal prompts, and photos. At that point, the book became very clear in my mind and I started to curate each week's theme, connecting my in-person classes to my on-demand classes, and parlaying my dharma talks into the written words you'll find here in this book.

I've learned a lot in this past year. I've relearned a lot as well. For me, like for everyone, a lot of things did not go as planned in 2020. I took a lot of time to plan classes, teach them in person, film them, edit them, download them, market them, and then repeat the process week after week.

I took a lot of time to read, study, watch webinars, and listen to podcasts. I even audited a two-hundred-hour yoga teacher training course! And something unexpected happened: I started to question a lot of my ideas and assumptions. In fact, I am still in the process of questioning some of my most deeply held beliefs. But I also realized that this process of simply asking why I'm saying or doing something has been transformational in my growth. And I know this transformation is not and may never be complete: I will continue to shift and change.

Out of respect and appreciation for the yoga practice, I stopped saying "Namaste" in my classes this year. I began having difficult conversations about cultural appropriation and appreciation. You can check out the *Yoga Girl* podcast: "Conversations from the Heart, Why I Stopped Saying 'Namaste' with Susanna Barkataki" (November 13, 2020) for further insights into why.

Part of the way through the year, I also shifted from giving "All Level" Vinyasa classes to specifying the level of the class. "One size fits all" doesn't seem to fit anyone, so I began to question whether "All Level" classes can fit anyone either. This change was inspired by Francesca Cervero's podcast, *The Mentor Sessions*.

As you take this journey with me, I ask you to remember that what I share is drawn from my own personal experience. Yoga is individual to each and every practitioner. Yoga is not a substitute for medical attention, examination, diagnosis, or treatment. I urge you to progress at your own pace. If you experience any pain or discomfort, listen to your body, adjust the posture, and ask for support. Continue to breathe smoothly. If at any point you feel overexertion or fatigue, please respect your body and mind and rest before continuing your yoga practice.

Finally, I don't have all the answers. As I said, I continue to learn and grow through my own yoga practice. But I hope these themes, prompts, and sequences that I have created for you will guide you to ask questions of yourself and your community, and enable you to shine both on and off the mat!

FOREWARD

In my line of work as an Integrative Health Practitioner, looking through the lens of Ayurveda, I see that stress has become a 'normal' part of daily life for most people. That could explain why so many Americans - about 16 million - have started taking yoga classes or doing yoga at home.

For those seeking a lasting cure for anxiety, or health issues and a greater sense of connectedness, yoga provides real and lasting benefits. This ancient system which is the sister science to Ayurveda connects body and mind through postures, breathing exercises and meditation. Yoga and Ayurveda take into account that body, mind and spirit must be in balance to achieve good health.

Many people report that yoga gives them an overall feeling of well-being. Research shows that yoga can help alleviate pain, and reduces stress. Studies show that yoga causes an increase in serotonin and dopamine - these are the body's natural pain killers and pleasure neurotransmitters. No wonder we feel so much better after yoga.

Another reason we feel so much better after a yoga practice is that cortisol levels are reduced, this is a hormone that the body releases in response to stress. There are many studies that point to high cortisol levels as being the culprit for stress, fatigue, chronic fatigue, adrenal fatigue and a host of immune imbalance.

If the potential health benefits of yoga aren't enough to make you want to try it, consider this: Yoga can also make you look more toned and fit and help you move with greater ease, especially as you age.

However, when we speak about healing and good health, we must look deeper and more fully at ourselves and our lifestyles than we generally do in this 'make it easy, make it quick, and make it something someone else does for me' society.

When I first met Veronique, it was clear that she had a message worth sharing. Veronique has her own personal story and her journey that ensued has taken her on a path of deep reflection.

Her purpose in writing this book is to share her discoveries as a seeker.

According to the Vedas, the ancient sacred scriptures of India, six qualities are necessary to succeed in any venture: proper effort, perseverance, courage; knowledge of the given pursuit; skill and resources; and the capacity to overcome obstacles. It is these qualities that have brought Veronique great success. I watched her daily routines become her daily discipline, I have seen the grace in Veronique's life increase. She has applied a constant alertness in her life. Her practice of yoga and asanas and meditation have allowed her to practice good health as part of her daily life.

What Veronique has done in this book is put those tools into an easy to follow primer so that you can utilize the very same tools she has used. This book is a synthesis of her life's discoveries. The un-erasable truths and knowledge that she found within herself that lie in each one of us.

We can all tap into this storehouse.

Although this book is based upon the yogic system of wellness, she has extracted many of her lessons from Ayurveda and other global practices. Each one of us has its own special practices or sadhanas. These are wholesome activities that are attuned to nature. This book takes you on an explorative year-long journey that is rooted in her personal experience. Veronique is indeed a shining yogi. Her true work has only just begun. And I take great joy in watching her wisdom open to others.

Shine On & Off the Mat will bring benefit to everyone who is conscious of personal health, our connected environment and wants the best path to health and happiness.

While yoga may not cure everything that ails you - it will help you manage stress more easily and guide your way to feeling more vibrant with increased vitality. And that can make a huge difference in your overall health. So, let's all take a deep cleansing breath and get started on our best path to overall health and happiness.

KERRY HARLING AYURVEDA PRACTITIONER, M.ED. CAP

CEO OF THE HOLISTIC HIGHWAY

UNIVERSITY OF PITTSBURGH'S CENTER FOR INTEGRATIVE MEDICINE

AUTHOR: THE 25-DAY AYURVEDA CLEANSE

OWNER OF TED TALK: WHY CONTEXT IS EVERYTHING IN HEALTH CARE

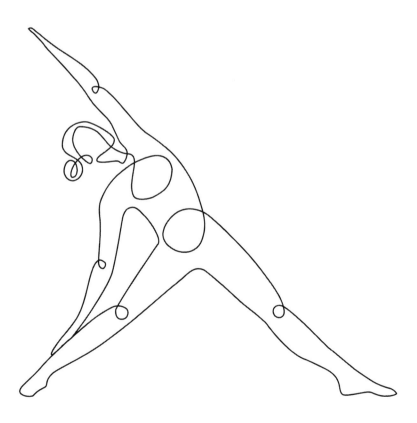

1. THEME: LET GO

When you realize the truth that everything changes, and find your composure in it, there you find yourself in nirvana.

—Suzuki Roshi

This has been an unprecedented time with coronavirus taking so many lives all over the world and disrupting others with grief and anxiety. We have watched our landscape transform around us, both socially and economically. Social distancing is still in place in many cities across the globe, necessitating new approaches in yoga instruction. Many classes now take place online. Some have closed down entirely. It's a scary and uncertain time, and many of us live in fear for our health and our financial future. If we can't go outside, we will take this opportunity to go inside.

Letting go is a beautiful way to arrive and arrive again in your yoga practice, disentangling yourself from the stresses of the surrounding world. It's a lifelong journey, letting go. I remember when I first began practicing yoga in the wake of Hurricane Sandy in NYC, I was drawn by a deep longing to let go. I was pursuing an acting career in New York, the city that never sleeps, and I was tense, stressed, and generally agitated most of the time. That first yoga class was perhaps the first time I took conscious breaths in my entire life. I knew I wanted to let go of the angst within me, but I didn't know how. I felt bombarded by drama and rejection daily, and it was slowly eating away at the creative soul that had motivated me to pursue the arts in the first place.

As I began moving my body and breathing regularly, the connection between setting an intention and letting go of the results really set in. Though I still yearned to one day practice "advanced" yoga poses, I shifted from feeling competitive or intimidated to feeling truly inspired.

So, this week, I am inviting you to let go, as best you can, as much as possible: of the unknown, of the what-ifs, of your uncertainties, of the things you can't control.

VIDEO: <u>Let Go</u>

PLAYLIST: <u>Let Go</u>

FEATURED SONG: <u>"Let Go" by Frou Frou</u>

HIGHLIGHTED POSE/TRANSITION: Cat pulling its tail. Through many twists and pretzel shapes, this is the shape we close practice with to illustrate how we can breathe when we feel like we're all tied up. We position ourselves in the ultimate twist in order to release and LET GO of those things we have no control over. I also love twists to detoxify the body and wring out the thoughts that are no longer serving.

JOURNAL PROMPT: *Name one to three things you can let go of this week.*

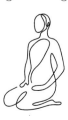

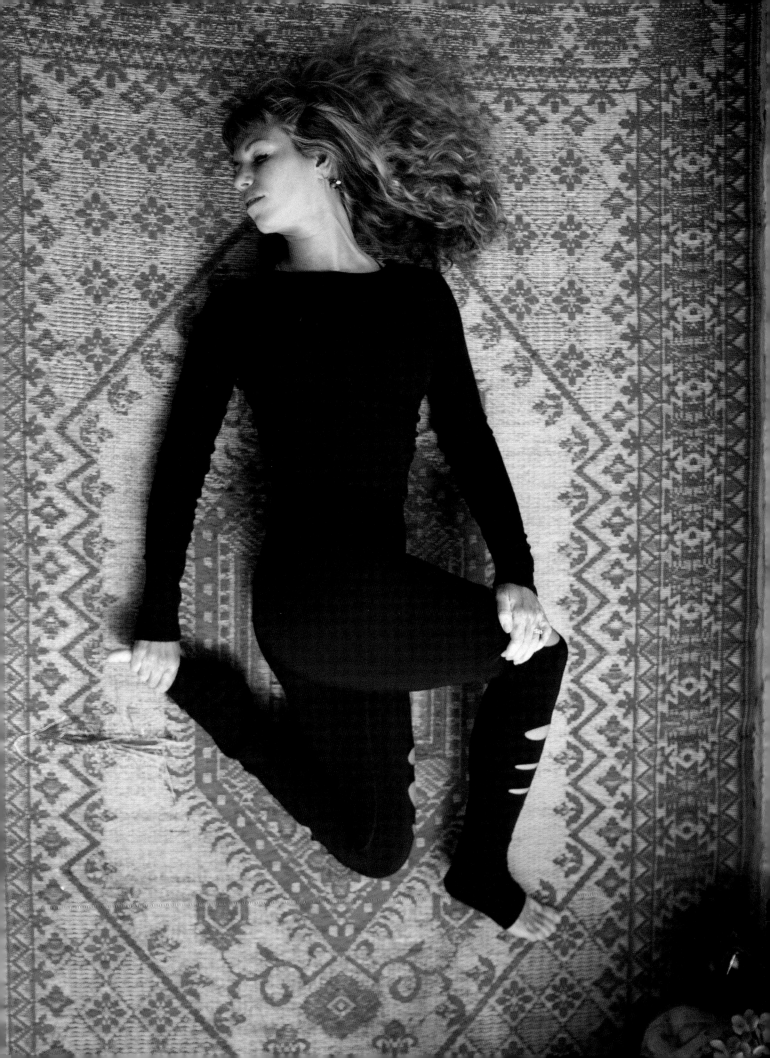

2. THEME: SLOWING DOWN

This universal message of slowing down has had a profound impact on me. The importance of slowing down, both in our yoga practice as well as away from the yoga mat, calls us to a heightened mindfulness.

This week, we will slow down our breath, slow down our thoughts, slow down our movements, and cultivate the practice of pausing to observe. This can be carried off the mat most specifically during those everyday activities we often think of as routine: eating, driving, running errands, immersing ourselves in media/social media, even engaging in in-person conversation. As we slow down, we can truly begin to cultivate an awareness of when we are actually fully conscious and present.

Slowing down has always been a challenging practice for me. I "thrived" for nine years in NYC, speed walking from point A to point B while simultaneously returning emails, running lines in my head for a play I was rehearsing, looking at people around me for character study, possibly grabbing a one-dollar pizza slice and pretending that was a meal, all while en route to the next thing. It was exhausting, but I won't deny I loved it! I loved the feeling of productivity! I loved the energy of a vibrant city! But I also knew very palpably that that level of energy, pace, and anxiety was not sustainable in the long term.

When I moved to Vero Beach, Florida, in June 2018, the entire pace of my existence shifted dramatically. I went from boasting about all the things I was doing, how much I was accomplishing simultaneously, to feeling grateful if I arrived fifteen minutes early to teach a yoga class so I could sit by the ocean and read a few pages of my book.

I'll be honest: I still love to feel productive and I can still get obsessed with my to-do lists sometimes (read: daily). As with letting go, the practice of slowing down is a lifelong practice.

Come into it slowly, mindfully, and with grace.

VIDEO: <u>Slowing Down</u>

PLAYLIST: <u>Let Go</u>

FEATURED SONG: <u>"You Can't Rush Your Healing" by Trevor Hall</u>

HIGHLIGHTED POSES/TRANSITIONS: The in-between poses/transitions such as slow motion entry and exit, from headstand through Vinyasas. I love to play with how slowly I can transition from one movement to another and to savor the in between. You can play with focusing on curiosity as you ask yourself, "Where am I feeling sensation here?"

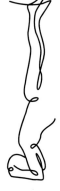

Be humble for you are made of earth. Be noble for you are made of stars.

—Serbian proverb

JOURNAL PROMPT: *Choose one activity you do on a daily basis and decide to do this one activity mindfully. For example, eat away from the TV or your smartphone.*

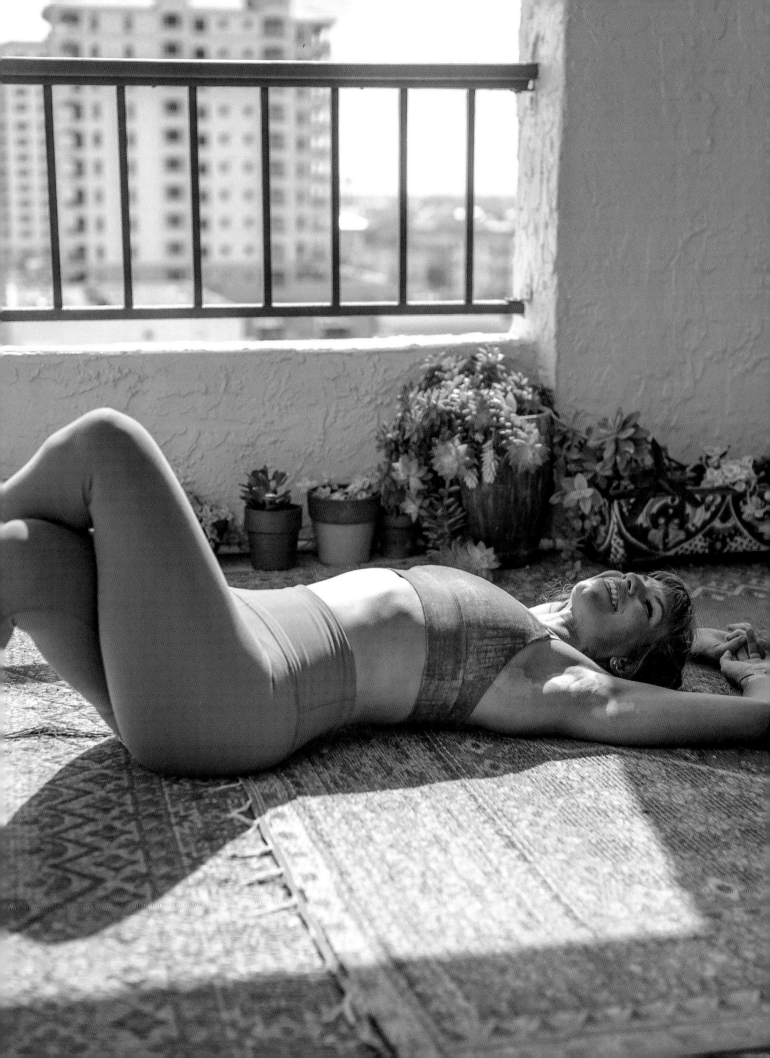

3. THEME: REFLECTION

Coming from letting go and slowing down, we move organically into our next phase: reflection. Observe your own thoughts from a space of curiosity, journal those thoughts that continue to reappear, and take this time and space to turn inward, using the opportunity to express, feel, create, explore, grow, and nurture. We all have a list of things we would do, "if only I had more time…" Each week, choose at least one item from your list and do it. Are there people, friends, or family, you have not spoken to in more than a month? Each week, choose one of these people to reach out to and check in with them. It's important to stay connected in any and all ways we can, especially when practicing social distancing.

We may be physically apart, but we can still connect. Finally, what brings you joy? Each day, do at least one thing that brings you joy. It could be anything, from yoga to walking in the park, to self-pampering routines, to a solo dance party in your living room, to curling up with a great book. This is one of the most rewarding ways to practice your yoga off the mat.

Inhale, exhale, repeat.

One of the projects from my own "if only I had more time…" list is my on-demand yoga series. I was in the hospital in the wake of Hurricane Dorian due to the stress of potentially losing our first house. Then, I was panicking about all the classes I would have to miss while recovering. It became very clear, amidst all the blood work and imaging the doctors were doing on me, how integral my health was to my being able to simply show up and teach each class. I literally don't have the stomach for all the fear-inducing media I was consuming at the time. I had gastritis (inflammation of the stomach), and it took more than nine months to fully heal.

In addition to feeling well, I also need to be fully present. I began to think about ways I could reach out beyond the traditional studio environment with my yoga practice and instruction. I am very passionate about making my yoga classes accessible for many reasons. I and many others relish the feeling of community offered by the yoga studio model, but that is not the experience for everyone. Many prefer taking classes at home, sometimes because they, for various reasons, feel uncomfortable in a group class setting, or because it's not feasible for them to arrange childcare, they have limited transportation options, there isn't a yoga studio nearby, or simply because physical or emotional considerations make being at home more comfortable.

I want to create yoga offerings for everybody.

VIDEO: <u>Reflection</u>
PLAYLIST: <u>Reflection</u>
FEATURED SONG: "<u>Terms of Surrender</u>" by Hiss Golden Messenger

HIGHLIGHTED POSES/TRANSITIONS: Begin practice in child's pose and end in corpse pose. Observe the journey and make peace with the legacy you leave behind. Embrace grace through all transitions despite the challenges that arise.

JOURNAL PROMPT: *At the end of this week, write down your favorite practice that brings you joy.*

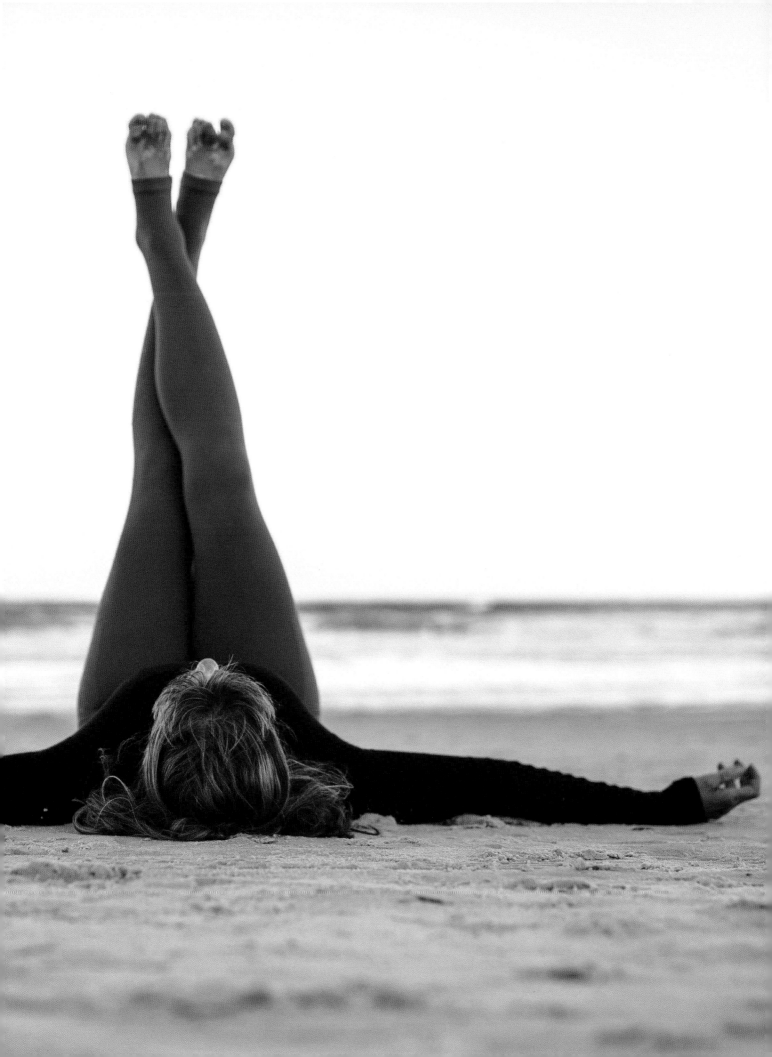

4. THEME: SELF-LOVE

I t's time for falling in love with yourself! Time alone is an invitation to get reacquainted with ourselves free from the distractions of the external world (or most of them, at least). What are the attributes of you that you love? What are the attributes of you that you don't love? Can you learn to get friendly and love them too? Or can you let those attributes go? As you inquire within, with compassion and understanding, claim this opportunity as your chance to grow, evolve, dig deeper, process, address, and take stock of what is serving and what is not. In this way, you can better differentiate between the internal and the external worlds. Are you in love with the way that you cope in times of stress—is it serving? Are you in love with the way you cope with change—is it serving?

How can you begin within and seek opportunity, rather than focusing on fear or restriction?

One of the best practices for self-love that I've discovered for myself is embarking on my Ayurveda journey. I signed up for a yearlong program through Holistic Highway as a step toward healing my gastritis (still unsettled nine months after Hurricane Dorian) and exploring this sister science of yoga to help heal my skin. Since 2000, I've had an autoimmune disease called vitiligo. According to the Mayo Clinic website, "Vitiligo is a condition in which the skin loses its pigment cells (melanocytes). This can result in discolored patches in different areas of the body, including the skin, hair and mucous membranes." There is no known cure.

I've spent ridiculous amounts of time and money at dermatologists, struggling to treat this disease topically. Finally in December 2019, I planned to get large tattoos on my feet of trees with intertwining branches like a watercolor painting. I yearned to claim power over my white spots and color them with art. I meditated on what my new feet would look like, and I even did a trial run with markers to see if I could get friendly with the idea of trees on my feet for the rest of my days in this body. I loved the reminder of grounding energy, but I continued to resist.

During this time, Ayurveda kept coming up in different conversations with friends and students, and at acupuncture. My initial thought was to find a meal delivery service for my specific dosha (metabolic type). This is how I discovered Holistic Highway in my research. I now see the power, not only of what we put into our body but also of all the beautiful morning rituals like tongue scraping, dry brushing, and self-massage with oil; mindfulness practices like eating consciously in combination with herbs; and sleeping the same hours each night. All play a role in my digestive and dermal health. Ultimately, this self-care practice is a deep healing practice. In just the first few months of my Ayurveda journey, my stomach feels fully healed and some of my white spots have begun to re-pigment.

VIDEO: <u>Self-Love</u>
PLAYLIST: <u>You Can't Rush Your Healing</u>
FEATURED SONG: <u>"You Can't Rush Your Healing" by Trevor Hall</u>

HIGHLIGHTED POSES/TRANSITIONS: Cat-cow with self-hug. You may practice articulating your spine seated. Begin seated, open your arms as you arch your spine for cow pose. Then, wrap your arms around yourself as you round your spine for cat pose.

In a gentle way, you can shake the world.

—Gandhi

JOURNAL PROMPT: *What are subtle or grand ways to express love to yourself? Circle just three of these and practice these this week.*

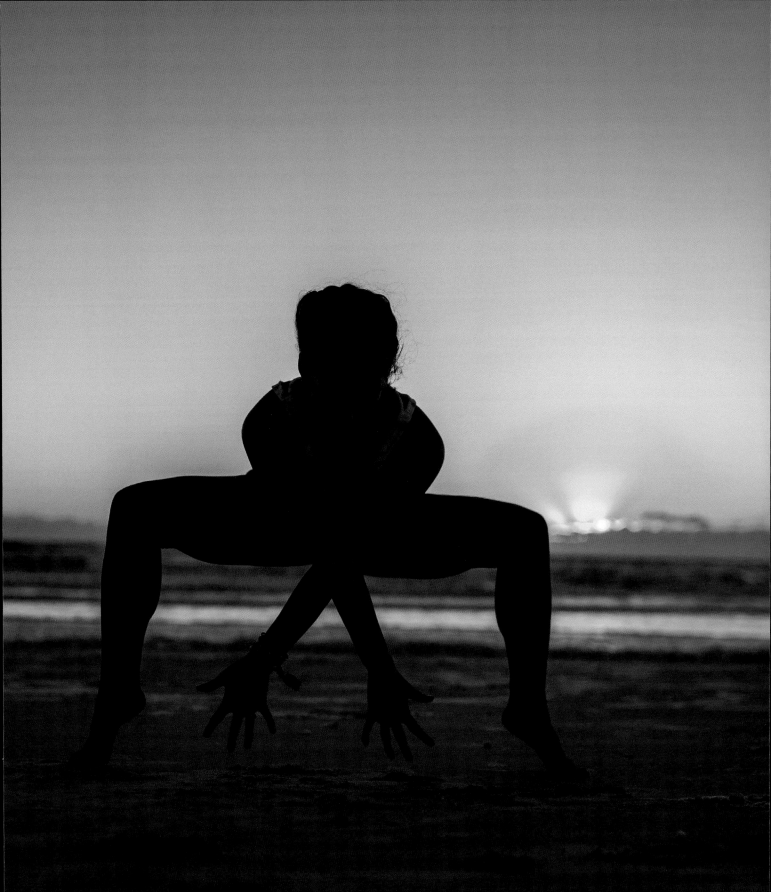

5. THEME: SPARK INSPIRATION

Create space in the body and the mind to find inspiration. Improvise in the flow, add different arm variations, or take a different kind of flow, all in the spirit of inviting space in the body and the mind to create inspiration from within. As we deepen our practice, my hope is that you shift from seeking inspiration outside of yourself to creating inspiration within. Get excited; feel the butterflies in your belly; make the hairs on your arms stand up!

When I move around on my mat and play, I'm always searching for unique variations of shapes and new pathways to transition, discovering new foundations to sequence toward a peak pose, in order to address a certain physical/emotional feeling, or to express the theme of the class. Then, I like to find songs and artists that resonate with the sequence and the message for each class.

Before the corona virus, I had seventeen group classes per week. Part of the inspiration for our explorations came from adjusting and shifting the same sequence throughout the week to align with the style of the class and who was there. No two classes were exactly the same.

Sometimes the energy in the room was chill and mellow, which would inspire me to adjust some of my planned standing poses so that they could be taken on the back instead. Sometimes the energy in the room was vibrant and energetic, which would inspire me to flow through the sequence, taking opportunities to echo select shapes in an inversion or arm balance. I truly relished observing how each class could develop these shifts and turns into a curated sequence week after week. My personal practice and my teaching style continue to evolve because of my students.

VIDEO: <u>Spark Inspiration</u>

PLAYLIST: <u>Inspiration</u>

FEATURED SONG: <u>"City of Stars" by Gavin James</u>

HIGHLIGHTED POSES/TRANSITIONS: Nontraditional Vinyasa, playful and unique variations of shapes and transitions. Standing forward fold with legs crisscrossed and as wide as the mat, turning around to find downward-facing dog facing the back of the mat. Downward-facing dog with cow-face legs.

The quieter the mind becomes, the more that you can hear.

—Ram Dass

JOURNAL PROMPT: *What inspires you, who inspires you, when are you inspired, and why are you inspired? And how can you create glimpses of profound inspiration daily for yourself? Start with yourself and then share it!*

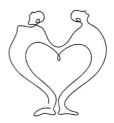

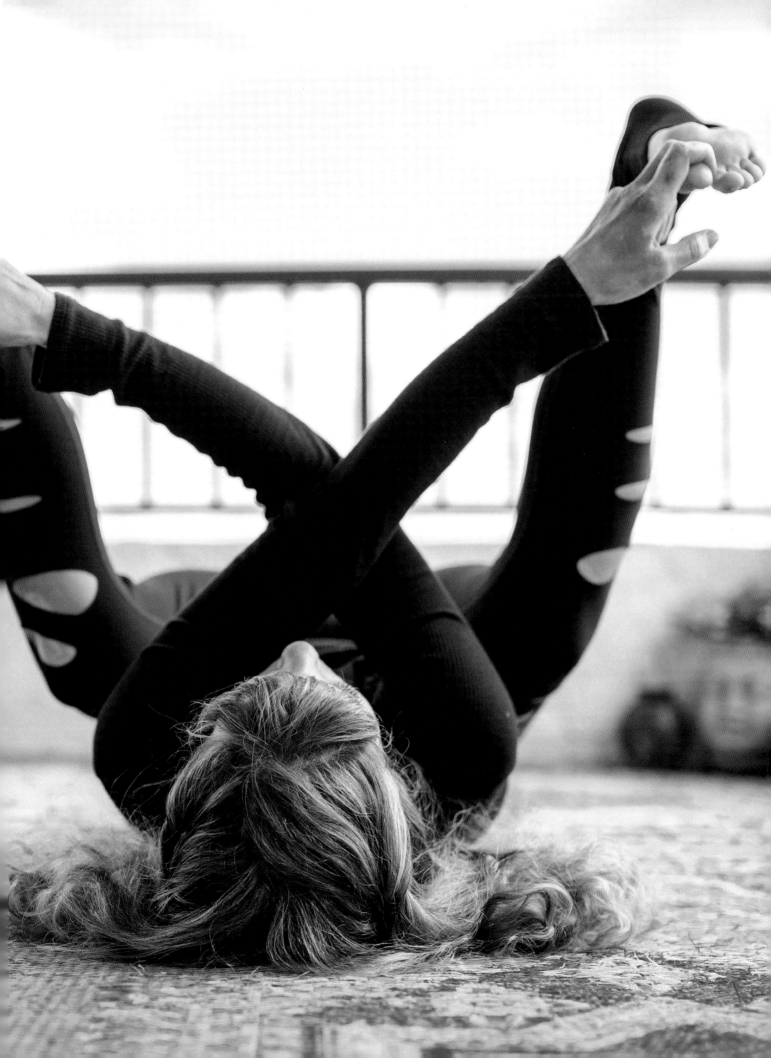

6. THEME: EMBRACE SILENCE

We can make our minds so like still water that beings gather about us that they may see, it may be, their own images, and so live for a moment with a clearer, perhaps even with a fiercer life because of our quiet.

—William Butler Yeats

What can be discovered in silence, and how can we become quiet in mind and body? The inspiration for this practice is to give space to answer questions that are on repeat in your mind; give space to feel each shape and give space to find comfort in the silence.

We habitually tend to fill time up with to-do lists, phone calls, or multitasking (or, at least, I know I do!), and the yoga practice is designed to quiet the mind. When we break up with these habits of moving quickly and doing too much at once, we can continue this practice of stillness/silence off the mat. What does it look like to drive without the distraction of music, news radio, or a podcast? How does it feel to sit in the same room with a loved one in silence? Rather than seeking to fill every moment with sound of some kind, when we become comfortable with silence, we discover a peacefulness that gives us the space to enter the mind and the body.

When the monkey mind continues to chatter on, consider cleaning your space. Clutter or unwanted items or an unmade bed can be very loud indeed. Start small and create one small space that is quiet in distractions as well as actual sound. Give your senses some repose and recommit to stillness. Then, embrace silence.

Some of my favorite memories of silence come from the early 2000s when I lived in Los Angeles. This was back when I was powered by coffee and could somehow function on just a few hours of sleep. I had started my own nonprofit theatre company called Athena Theatre when I was twenty-two years old, and I was giving it everything I had. I discovered that after 11:00 p.m. was the best time to get things done because the quiet of the night set in, the emails ceased to flood my inbox, and my mind felt clearer. My friend Kevin would come over and we would often have all-night work sessions. He would be on his laptop and I would be on mine and we would sit, quietly immersed in our respective passions: he with his computer programming and rocket science, and I with all the behind-the-scenes administrative work it takes to operate a theatre company. Sure, it wasn't the sort of silent meditation one engages in while sitting on a pillow, clearing the mind of distractions, but it really did feel meditative. Sitting at my desk at all hours, in a small apartment in Los Angeles, submerged in one singular focus, I surely felt at peace.

VIDEO: <u>Embrace Silence</u>

PLAYLIST: <u>Silence</u> (OR NO PLAYLIST AT ALL)

FEATURED SONG: <u>"A Moment of Silence" by The Neighbourhood</u>

HIGHLIGHTED POSE/TRANSITION: Holding asanas in silence

JOURNAL PROMPT: *Set a timer for five minutes and sit in silence. Then, write down all the thoughts that came through. Read what you wrote down and observe the thoughts without judgment. Then, let them go. Maybe tear this page out of your journal and burn it, or refer back to it if you'd like to make this a continuous practice and would find it useful to refer back to what thoughts reoccur.*

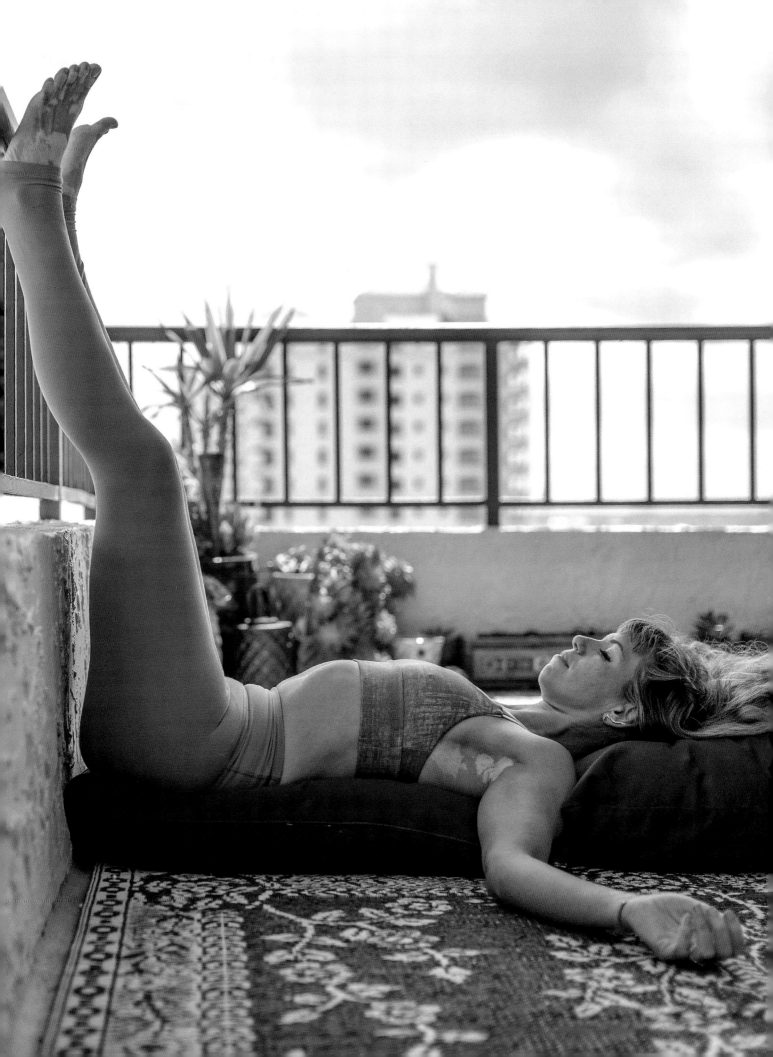

7. THEME: GRATITUDE

I often hear these days, "I can't wait until things go back to normal." I wonder how often we spend our days wishing things were different and waiting for certain moments to pass. If we can practice gratitude even though things are not exactly as we wish them to be—and perhaps especially because they are not perfect!—we can start to find a deeper peace in the present moment. So we flow through challenging shapes as a mirror of our breathing into challenging situations, remembering that the asana practice is intended to express these shapes as portals into the self, and practice the cessation of the fluctuations of the mind. How do we express gratitude when taking a shape on our injured side? How do we express gratitude when our livelihoods are taken away, or our loved ones are sick, or we are struggling? There is always something to be learned and compassion to be expressed. We can always continue to grow, practice strength and flexibility, and, at the same time, have a deep appreciation for what is. There is a teacher that lives in all things. When your mind becomes caught up in yearning for the past or the future, gently guide yourself toward a gratitude meditation. You can name what you are grateful for with each breath—whether in movement or stillness on the mat and extend this gratitude practice off the mat as well.

When there is time and space, I like to practice gratitude for the hard conversations and the relationships that ended badly, and to practice shifting from holding resentment to feeling the opportunity to learn and grow. I've had a lot of learning and growing to do! When I first moved to NYC, I had already spent nine years producing and acting in plays. I was excited to shift from producing published plays to developing new works. I met a playwright who, upon having many conversations surrounding the development of his play, decided to create a role for me. I was very excited for the opportunity, especially because he had connections to highly regarded industry types I knew would be coming to the staged reading. My company produced the reading with the understanding that we would stay on as producers when/if the play got picked up for a full production. However, after the reading, this playwright said he no longer saw me in the role and stopped returning my calls. The ironic thing was that he wrote the role for me! I was livid and felt betrayed and used. I had believed we were friends and I had trusted him, which had led me to make the one-time-only mistake of not drawing up a contract, which meant I had no legal recourse or protection. I was out-of-my-mind angry with him and with myself. The collapse of this relationship/production took me a while to process and get out of my system. To be honest, even now, writing this out, I feel my heart picking up pace. Ultimately, though I have learned to cultivate and embrace a sense of gratitude for this situation. Yes, the practical lesson is to always draw up contracts in working relationships, but the larger spiritual lesson to me is to practice nonattachment. I recognize now that when I do something and release my expectation of a certain result, I feel gratitude for simply having done the work at all.

VIDEO: <u>Gratitude</u>

PLAYLIST: <u>Gratitude</u>

FEATURED SONG: <u>"All My Days" by Alexi Murdoch</u>

HIGHLIGHTED POSE/TRANSITION: Butterfly seat with prayer hands as a double gratitude gesture of sorts. We flow with Anjali Mudra as a reminder to express gratitude through challenges, despite wanting things to be different.

JOURNAL PROMPT: *Write down all the people, places, and things you are grateful for.*

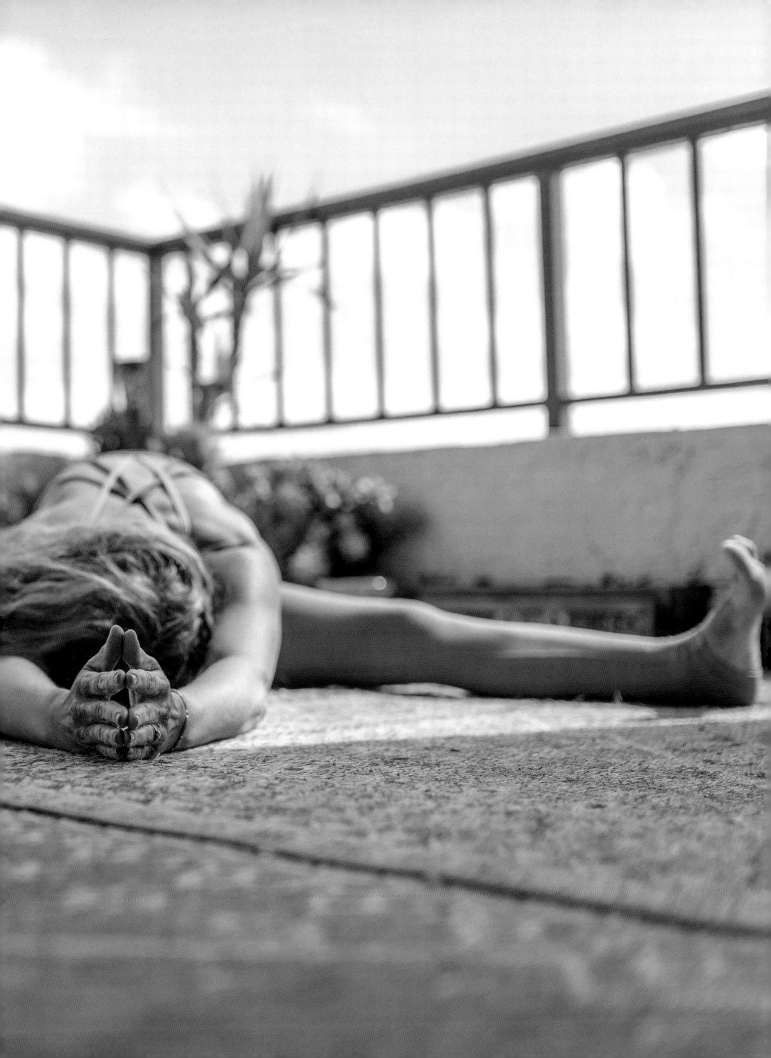

8. THEME: FINDING TRUTH

How do we unpack what we know to be true? How do we know whether our belief in ourselves and others is real? Take a step back and observe whether you have any beliefs that may be limiting you. Ask yourself whether those beliefs are based in truth or fear. Do you often find yourself saying, "I can't do this or that or I'll never be able to _____?" These thoughts are very powerful and become stories we tell ourselves and beliefs we manifest, whether based in truth or fear. For example, imagine you once suffered an injury to your right knee and have spent years telling yourself and your yoga instructors, "I can't do this pose or that pose."

You're right.

But imagine, for a moment, that you instead show up to your mat with a beginner's mind, without deciding for your knee what its limitations are, and you try one of the forbidden shapes. Just for a breath. Then, the next practice you try for two breaths, and so on. When practicing mindfully, over time, a healing will transpire. Yes, your knee will be able to move in ways you thought were impossible and, more profoundly, your mind is opening up to all the possibilities that you previously thought were impossible. There is a distinct difference between opting out of what you believe you cannot do and guiding yourself to live and rediscover the true you.

I actually have chronic pain in my right knee and right ankle. I dislocated my ankle during a performance of *Wait until Dark*. I was playing Susy Hendrix (the blind character played by Audrey Hepburn in the film adaptation). One fateful evening, during the climactic fight scene, the antagonist accidentally fell on my leg and I actually felt my kneecap come out. When I managed to stand up, it popped back into place. I hobbled around for a day or two, believing it would heal on its own, but it didn't, and I ended up spending years in and out of physical therapy. As if that wasn't bad enough, on my way to one of those sessions, I missed a step on the staircase in the hospital and badly sprained my ankle. I feel very fortunate that the biggest complaint I have is that these injuries make lotus and hero's poses quite uncomfortable. And yet it really irks me. But I am learning to let go of these injuries. And when I properly warm up and have the necessary props for support, I do indeed witness that the limitations I put on my body can slowly open up.

VIDEO: <u>Finding Truth</u>

PLAYLIST: <u>Patience</u>

FEATURED SONG: <u>"Because" by the Beatles</u>

HIGHLIGHTED POSES/TRANSITIONS: Twists! Peak pose: single-legged chair pose with eagle arms with twist.

JOURNAL PROMPT: *What is a false truth you often tell yourself that you are ready to let go of? Now rewrite that phrase as truth. For example, rewrite "My balance is horrible" to "I breathe into the balance I have."*

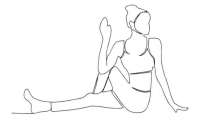

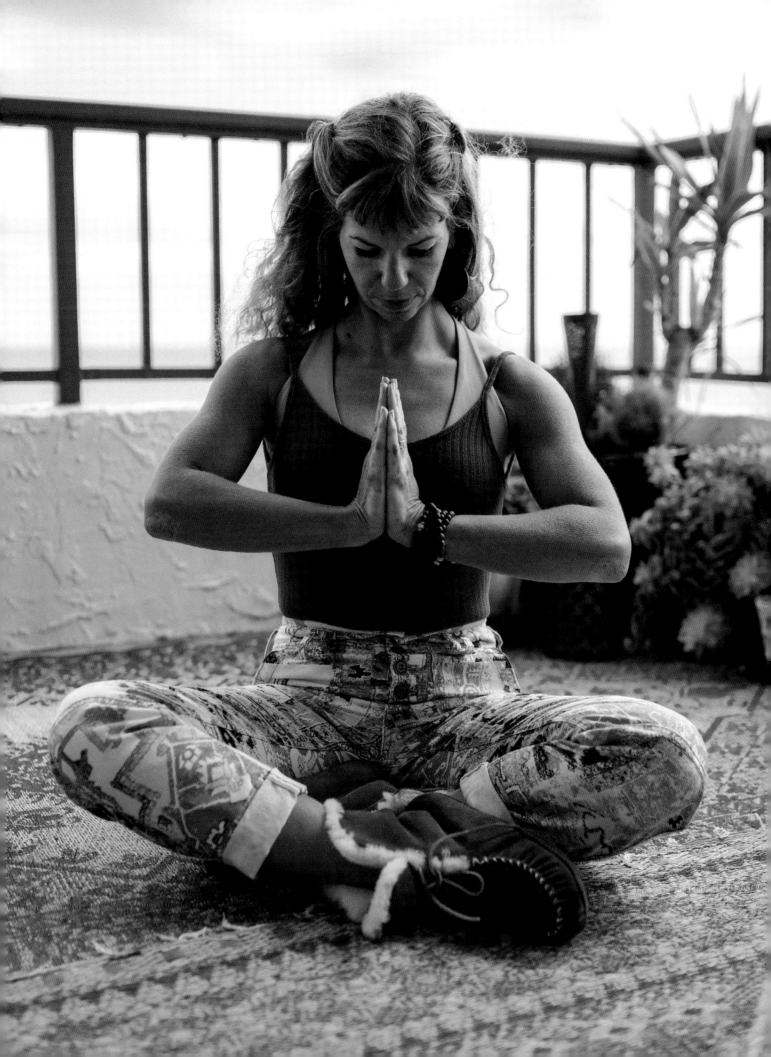

9. THEME: FLOW WITH GRACE

Today's theme was inspired by a recent journal prompt I came across to name three people I admire and next to each name list three qualities I admire about each person. One person I admire is Audrey Hepburn and one quality I admire about her is grace. It is said that each of us possesses every quality in those we admire and by embodying these qualities, we can achieve the best version of ourselves. So, with this prompt, I invite you to embody grace—however that resonates for you. This could appear as breathing more fluidly, moving like peaceful water, or embracing stillness with a sense of ease in both the mind and the body. For me, I love finding fluidity in the arms, expressing more opening across the heart, landing lightly into the feet. One of my favorite transitions is from Warrior III into Crescent Lunge, where I try to land the back foot down as slowly as possible and then express victory in the arms when I do. It's a powerful practice to find grace within each thought, each breath, each word, each movement/action. What does that look and feel like for you? Does grace come easily to you or is it more of a challenge? Why? (It's not the official journal prompt for this week, but consider writing a journal entry about how grace sits with you.) Take a look and keep coming back to the practice of flowing with grace. With practice, grace will become your own.

When I was a little girl, I would often put on "concerts" for my grandparents in their living room. My grandfather bought me an Elvis Presley microphone and connected it to their double tape deck, recording each show. My number one requested song (from my grandparents) was "Somewhere over the Rainbow" from *The Wizard of Oz*. I thought at the time that my voice was on par with Judy Garland's because my family oooh'd and ahhhh'd whenever I sang. These living room concerts catalogue my singing when I was five through fifteen years old. During these years, I envisioned myself in movies or on a stage performing with the grace of Audrey Hepburn and the voice of Judy Garland. Let's just say that no one would cast me in a professional singing role outside of my imagination. I went on to perform many non-singing roles, however.

I revisit this memory because it brings me back to how what we do feels in our bodies. Let go of how it sounds or how it looks—how does it feel?! I still love to sing with the essence of Judy Garland in my mind. And I still love to move my body with the embodiment of Audrey Hepburn in my heart. It's the feeling that resonates with me. That's the beating of my soul.

VIDEO: <u>Flow with Grace</u>

PLAYLIST: <u>Hope</u>

FEATURED SONG: <u>"Don't Let Me Down" by Joy Williams</u>

HIGHLIGHTED POSES/TRANSITIONS: Equal part breath, flowing arms from volcano pose to standing forward fold and including flowing arms flow in low/high lunge.

JOURNAL PROMPT: *Name three people you admire and next to each name list three qualities you admire about each person.*

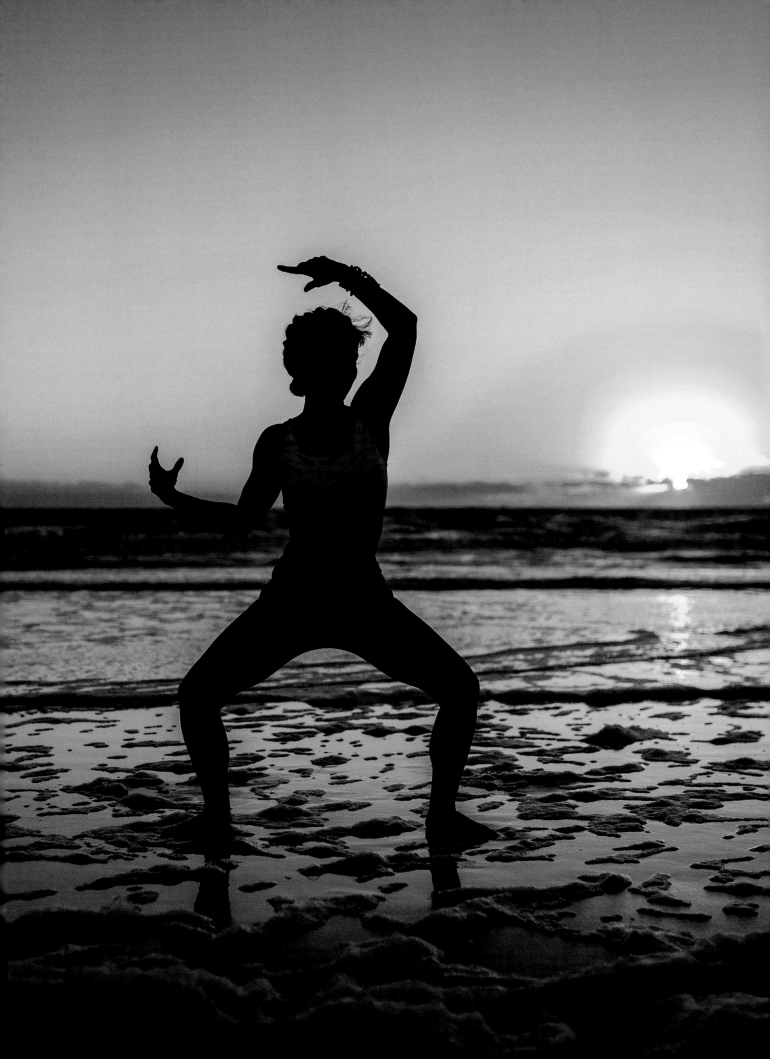

10. THEME: YOU ARE POWERFUL

Feeling powerful and being powerful may or may not be connected. What makes the mind feel powerful? What impedes that feeling? What role does posture play in the mind's perception of itself? I'm reminded of Amy Cuddy's TED talk on embodying powerful positions and the role they play in how we feel about ourselves. In this yoga practice, I invite you to examine when your mind is taking control and when you are in control of your thoughts. Additionally, how readily do you take child's pose, or modify it, and when do you embrace your strength (whether in cultivation or actual) and challenge yourself beyond what you think you can do? This is not about skipping rest and not modifying ever, but rather taking a look at when you embrace your power and whether you find yourself readily giving in at the first sign of challenge. You. Are. Powerful. This practice is intended to empower you with your breath, with your thoughts, with your words, and in your body.

When I meditate on a model for strength, I think of my grandmother, my dad's mom. She survived a lot! When she was a young girl, she and her mom were sent to Auschwitz. One day, my grandmother and her mom were taken to the gas chamber under the pretense that they were going to have a shower. At the last minute, the guards discovered the showers were broken. Their lives were spared. I get chills when I think about that day. I try to think of my Hungarian grandmother as a little girl just trying to stay alive, facing death every day simply because she happened to be born Jewish.

When my dad was ten years old, my grandparents decided to emigrate to Montreal. They came on a boat with just the clothes on their backs to build a better life for my dad. My grandma fought for her little family. Then, when I was born, she fought for me too. She had a fire in her belly that drove her to move mountains for anyone she loved. Being around that kind of strength is equal parts comforting and empowering. As my grandmother got older, dementia began to take over her mind. We had to move her to an assisted living facility so someone could monitor her medications. In the final years of her life, there were times she didn't recognize my dad and me. On our final visit we had been sitting around the kitchen table for about thirty minutes when she turned to me and asked in her thick Hungarian accent, "I don't know why your dad don't call me."

I said, "He's right here."

She said, "I don't know that. This old man is my son?"

My dad and I laughed with tears in our eyes because we knew we were forever young in her eyes. It was time for us to be strong and to practice patience with her as she asked the same question a million times just like we did as children. I don't know if I'll ever be as strong as my grandma was, but I certainly feel more powerful when I think of her.

VIDEO: <u>You Are Powerful</u>

PLAYLIST: <u>First Impressions</u>

FEATURED SONG: <u>"Where Is My Mind?" by Maxence Cyrin</u>

HIGHLIGHTED POSES/TRANSITIONS: Chair pose flow with block in between the thighs.

JOURNAL PROMPT: *What actions make you feel the most powerful?*

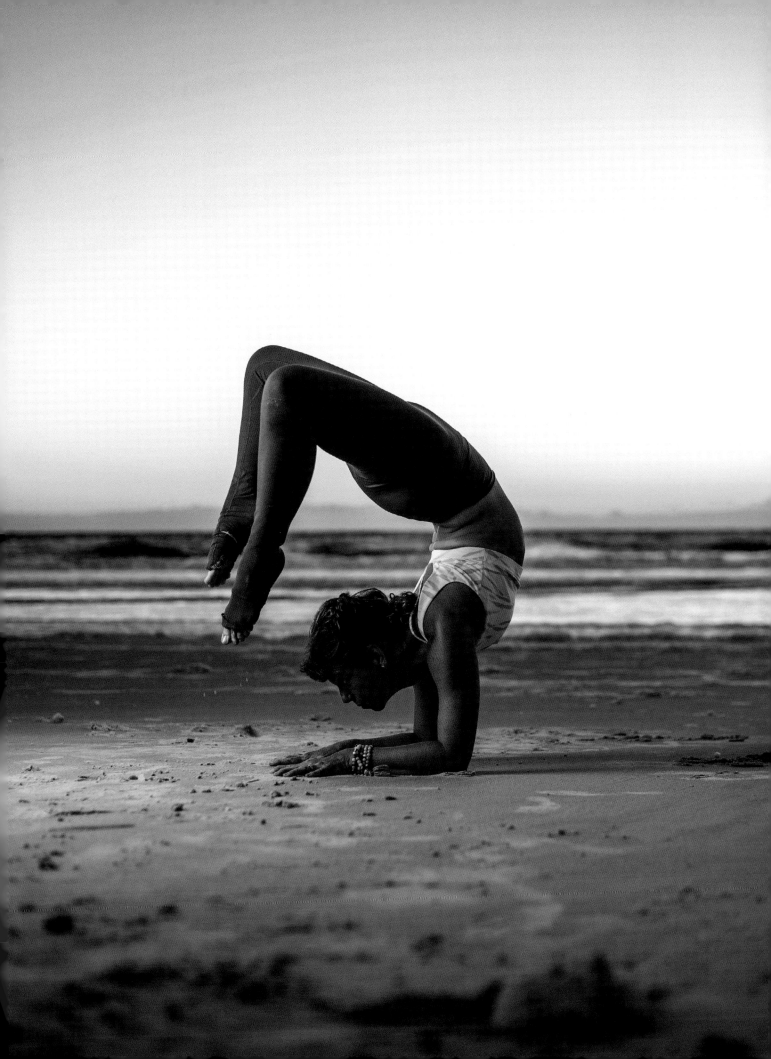

11. THEME: FORGIVENESS

Forgiveness for yourself and forgiveness for others: which one (if not both) are you holding back on offering? Without forgiveness, we remain in the past, feeling regret, hurt, betrayal, anger, and fear, and these emotions prevent us from fully arriving in the here and now. So this week's practice is an opportunity to tap into any unresolved relationships you may have with others or yourself and express forgiveness—not necessarily because it is earned, but because it brings you peace. The practice is designed to help you tune inward and find a space of reflection, and to open up a space where you can feel free. In this way, we can recognize and honor the surrender and fragility of forgiveness, as well as the strength and bravery.

I struggle with this one a lot.

My astrological sign is Scorpio, and I'm also my grandmother's granddaughter. I am extremely passionate and determined, I would readily forgo many of life's essentials for the sake of those I love. Perhaps it is because I crack my heart open so fully and so freely that I struggle with forgiveness when I feel my love is being taken advantage of. So I invite you to practice forgiveness with humility.

Maya Angelou has a great quote that I keep coming back to when I struggle with forgiveness: "It's one of the greatest gifts you can give yourself, to forgive. Forgive everybody."

This really hits home for me, and helps with the healing. Ultimately, it's not about them, the people who crossed us. Our forgiveness cannot be contingent on them apologizing. I sometimes have a war in my head about this. "If they would just admit that what they did was hurtful…or if we could just have a conversation to get to a resolution…" I've had these conversations. I've let my mind retell, relive, and reignite all of the pain over and over again. I like to take time to think about what's happened, journal about it, and hash it out again with a loved one. And then, as best as I can, I let it go for myself, not for them. Yes, there may be a glimmer of stubbornness that can't forget, but I try to let that be a lesson for myself going forward.

VIDEO: <u>Forgiveness</u>
PLAYLIST: <u>Humble Me</u>
FEATURED SONG: <u>"Forgive" by Trevor Hall, Luke Lesson</u>

HIGHLIGHTED POSE/TRANSITION: Humble Warrior.

JOURNAL PROMPT: *If you are ready, write down the name of the person you are ready to forgive. Write this person a letter letting them know you forgive them.*

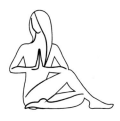

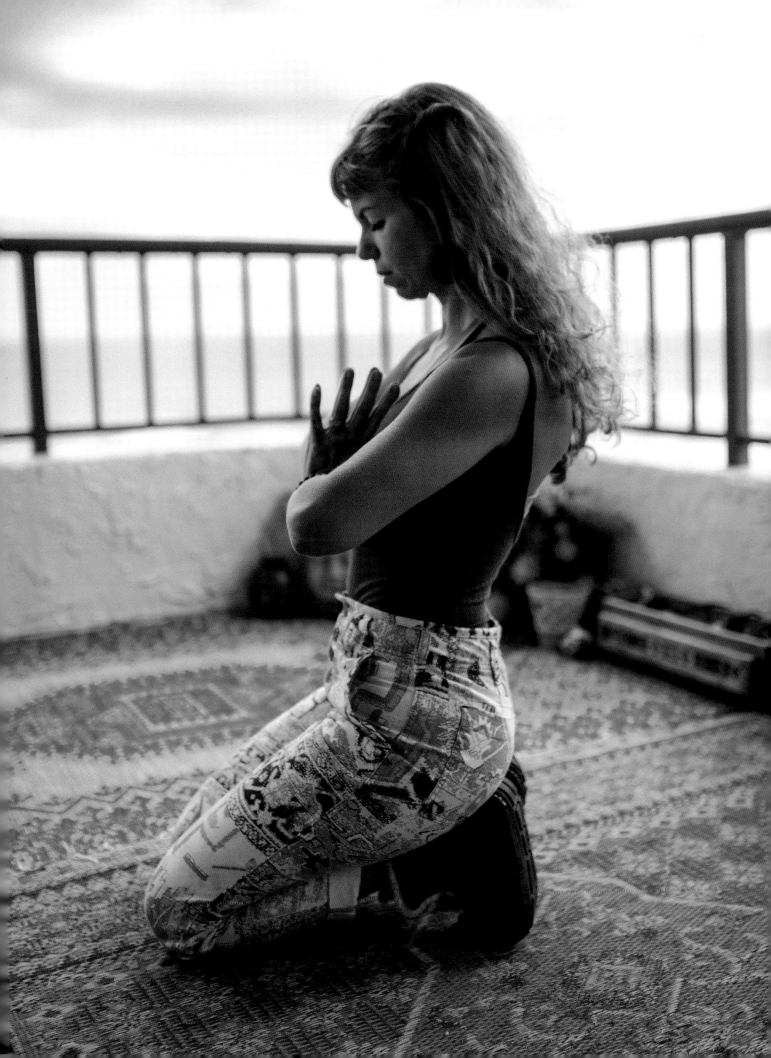

12. THEME: UNIVERSE IS ME

May all beings everywhere be happy and free, and may the thoughts, words, and actions of our lives contribute in some way to that happiness and freedom for all. The thoughts we have connect to the words we use and the actions we take. Starting with our own belief system of how we see ourselves and others, and see ourselves in others, we can shift from the "us vs. them" mentality. Have compassion with your thoughts; observe them in a space of curiosity and with a beginner's mind. What unites us is greater than what divides us.

Start within in meditation, in stillness or movement, and consider how you can show up in the world for social justice. I invite you to carry your yoga practice off the mat, embracing the yoga teachings of ahimsa (nonviolence) and union. Lead by example.

When I was in college, my parents initiated a conversation of acceptance with me. Both of them called and said something to the effect of, "I wanted to let you know that no matter who you are dating, no matter their race, religion, gender, as long as you're happy, that's all that matters." I remember thinking, "Wow, my parents are amazing!" I don't know what prompted their independent reaching out to give me their blessing to connect with any and all souls that inspire me without parameters, but I'm grateful they did. Connecting with all beings is an integral part of my own yoga practice. Sometimes, when I practice, I like to think of all the souls around the world that are simultaneously taking mindful breaths. There is a deep sense of connection when we practice in the same room, in a community space, and even when we tap into it while apart.

VIDEO: <u>Universe Is Me</u>

PLAYLIST: <u>Opening</u>

FEATURED SONG: <u>"Across the Universe" by Fiona Apple</u>

HIGHLIGHTED POSE/TRANSITION: Flow with hooked thumbs—connection within ourselves first, so that we can connect with others regardless of race, gender, sexuality, or beliefs.

JOURNAL PROMPT: *What actions can you take this week with the intention of universal connection to all?*

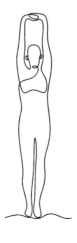

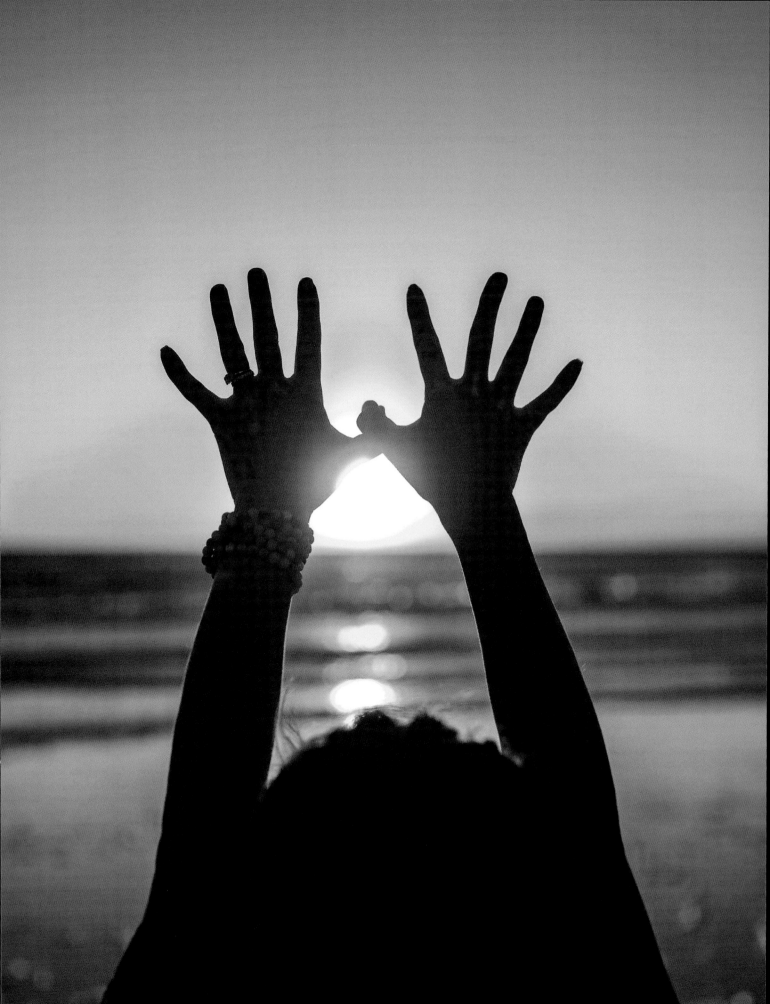

13. THEME: FOREVER GROWING

Nothing ever goes away until it teaches us that we need to learn.

—Pema Chödrön

When we are forever growing, we continually evolve and thrive. Perhaps the portal to growth is looking at how we can grow within the asana practice—showing up consistently and practicing shapes that challenge us. Perhaps the portal to growth is allowing the asana practice to be a moving meditation wherein we contemplate what we are striving to learn. We can allow the yoga practice to inspire us to always stay curious, challenge our previous beliefs, and strive to be the best version of ourselves every single day. Some days we may falter, feel tired, or feel blue. This is also a part of the growth journey, listening to your body and mind and being able to discern for yourself when it is appropriate to take rest and when it is necessary to push through the challenges. The objective of this theme is to start within and thereby be an inspiration to others.

I invite you to create space for yourself to keep learning. Dive into the subjects that excite you. And also stay open to how you're learning and maybe even unlearn some things (with humility) along the way.

VIDEO: <u>Forever Growing</u>

PLAYLIST: <u>The Garden</u>

FEATURED SONG: <u>"The Garden" by Jelani Aryeh</u>

HIGHLIGHTED POSE/TRANSITION: Tree pose in side plank.

JOURNAL PROMPT: *"I've always wanted to learn…" Take the first step this week to cultivate the knowledge you seek.*

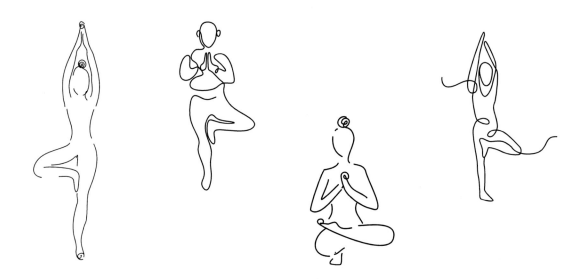

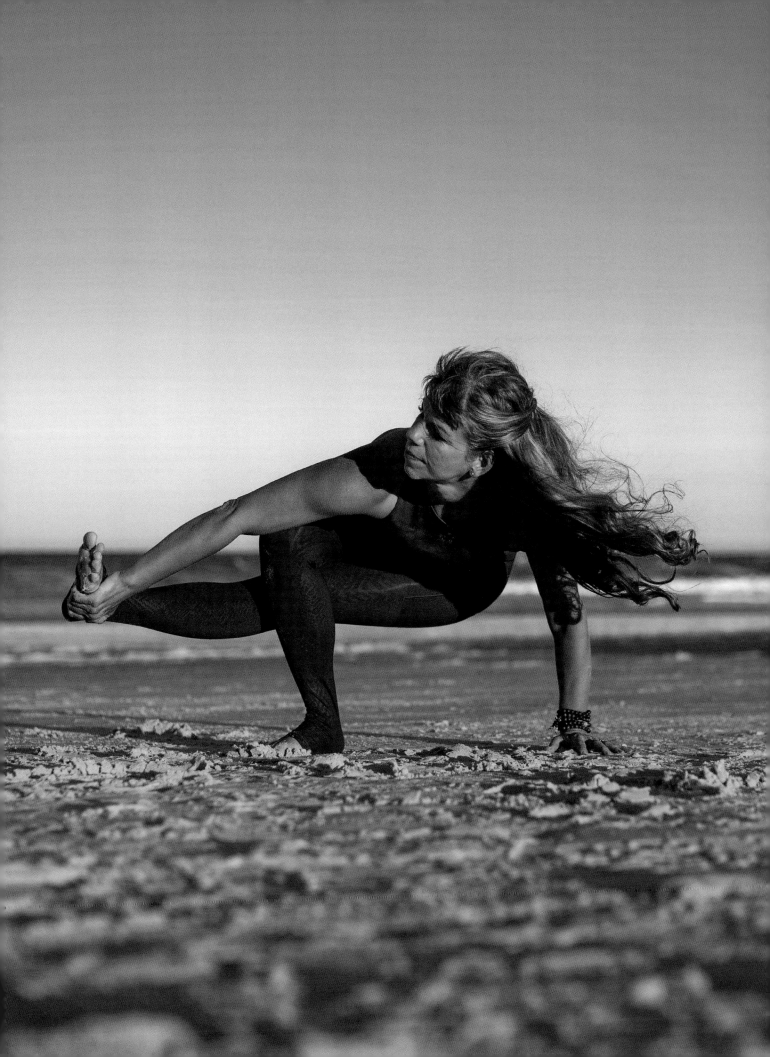

14. THEME: INTUITION EMERGES

When your intuition emerges, how do you respond? Are you one to follow your intuition, or do you second-guess, or let your brain override your gut? Are you also asking yourself how it adheres to Buddha's law: "Is it true? Is it kind? Is it necessary?" With your attention on your third eye center, we can focus your awareness onto that space of intuition and observe. Does a situation or a person leave you biting your tongue, stopping yourself from speaking your truth/following your intuitions? Why? Perhaps there isn't necessarily a shift, but try to cultivate an awareness of when and how you're silencing yourself, and ask yourself, "Is that serving?" Are your thoughts, words, and actions congruent with how you're visualizing yourself, and ultimately guiding yourself to emerge from a space of trust?

When I was fifteen years old, I decided to move to Scottsdale, Arizona, to live with my dad and stepmom and finish high school there. My parents had separated when I was young, but they are still good friends to this day. In my early teen years, I had begun visiting my dad and stepmom during school holidays and we grew closer while I lived with my mom in a suburb of Albany, New York. I think this spurred my decision to live with my dad as a "last chance" before going away to college. Looking back, it feels surprising that I would uproot myself, disrupt my schooling, and leave my friends from childhood to start anew as a high school junior. I return to this pivotal shift in my trajectory often. I can point to this move as one of the momentous intuitive decisions that shaped me into the person I am today. I shifted from being mostly a B student to an A student. I joined the swim team and befriended several people who had just moved to Arizona as well. One girl said she met with the guidance counselor, who said she could graduate early. I was intrigued, so I too visited the guidance counselor and I was also able to graduate a year early. I decided to move back to Upstate New York because I was familiar with Russell Sage College. As a teenager, I took voice, acting, and movement classes at the New York State Theatre Institute on the college's campus. Since I was just sixteen years old when I began college, I wanted to go somewhere familiar. The connections I made in college brought me to Los Angeles, where I founded my theatre company, which eventually brought me to NYC, which brought me to my yoga practice.

VIDEO: <u>Intuition Emerges</u>

PLAYLIST: <u>Inspiration</u>

FEATURED SONG: <u>"One Step Forward" by Direct</u>

HIGHLIGHTED POSE/TRANSITION: Child's pose with attention to third eye on the earth.

JOURNAL PROMPT: *Name a current or recent situation where you know in your gut what is right, but the mind or circumstance has left you second-guessing yourself. Now write from imagination how this plays out when you follow your intuition. Sometimes writing it out can release inhibiting factors, or maybe the simple act of writing it out can free you from the angst and worry surrounding this situation.*

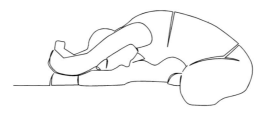

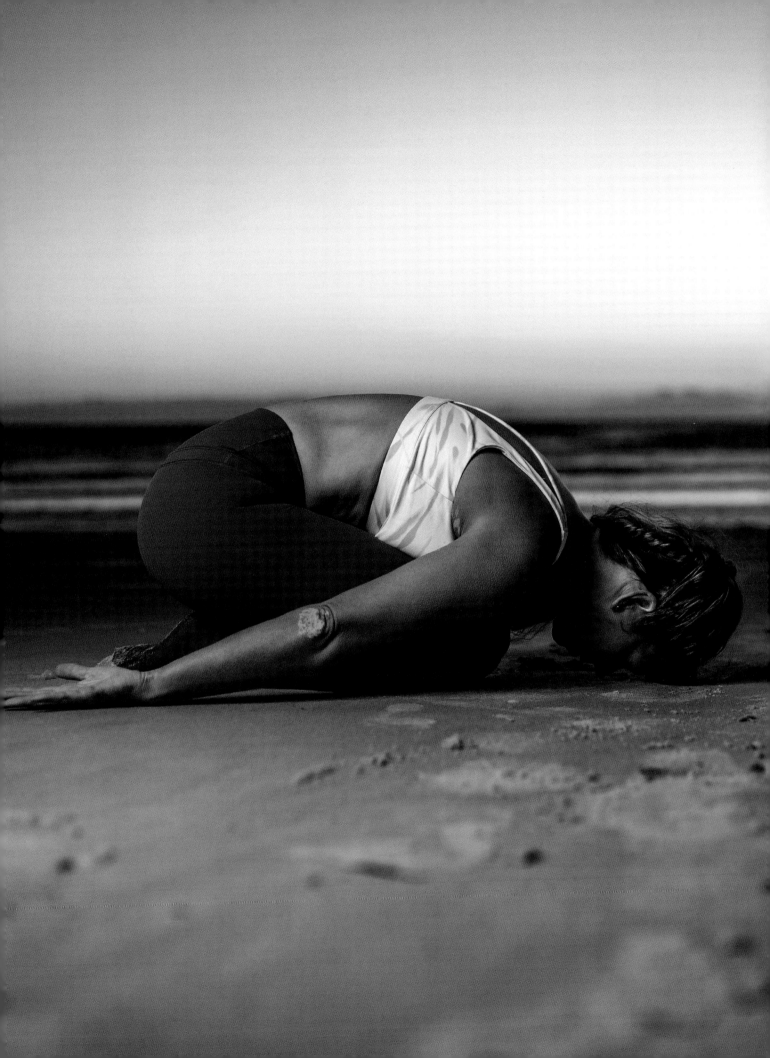

15. THEME: CLEANSE & RESET

began a cleanse this week and was inspired to let this inform my classes. When we think of a cleanse, we often think of some kind of adjustment to what we eat. Cleansing can go much deeper than the foods and drinks we put in our bodies, although adjusting our diet is a part of it. Cleansing extends to what we put on our skin, as well as self-care rituals that promote clean hygiene, using products that are cruelty free and free of chemicals. We can also look at how we maintain our home space, the habits we have that serve versus those that are in opposition to our well-being, and perhaps our relationships with those we surround ourselves with who inspire and allow us to be the best versions of ourselves versus those who don't. So as we practice with twists, think about one or two aspects of your life that you can let go of. Start with something fairly easy to give up or cut down on and see how you feel. Observe the habits and rituals that allow your light to shine and cultivate more of this abundance into your everyday life.

This past year I have cleansed in many ways. I eliminated coffee! This is a huge one for me, and I honestly would never have sought it out. I LOVE coffee and truly loved my morning coffee ritual. But the truth is that coffee doesn't agree with my body. So I've now tried to get friendly with the idea of being a tea drinker. I'm now also a mostly gluten-free, alcohol-free, and sugar-free vegan, and I try to eat local, fresh, and organic foods. I can on occasion eat or drink outside of my Ayurveda program, but I know in my gut (literally!) that I feel so much clearer when I eat clean. It's a journey of mindfulness practice and I'm only human. That said, I can have a treat every now and again, or even have wine and cheese as a celebration, and choose not to feel guilty about it.

I also gave away a lot of clothes I was no longer wearing, or some pieces that perhaps I wore only a few times. My friends and I did a clothing swap and then we donated all the clothes left over. It was a fun way to "shop" within our friend circle and provided the impetus we needed to let go of the extras in our respective closets.

The other ritual I implemented this year was a mind cleanse every Sunday. For twenty-four hours, I abstain from social media, I wash the towels and the sheets, and I take an Epsom salt bath. While I'm soaking, I do a face masque, wear cucumber slices, and listen to a guided meditation. I give myself a mani-pedi and then carry on with my daily ritual of oils and lotions for my face and body. I truly feel so peaceful and entirely cleansed closing the week in this way!

VIDEO: <u>Cleanse and Reset</u>

PLAYLIST: <u>The Garden</u>

FEATURED SONG: <u>"breathe again" by Joy Oladokun</u>

HIGHLIGHTED POSE/TRANSITION: Twisting it out to release the toxins in the body and let go of thoughts that aren't serving.

JOURNAL PROMPT: *Choose one thing you're ready to cleanse yourself of this week. This could be that late night snack, alcohol, or processed food. It could also be extra clutter on your desk or that junk drawer you've been meaning to get to. It could be obsessing about news or social media. It could be negative self-talk or getting wrapped up in gossip.*

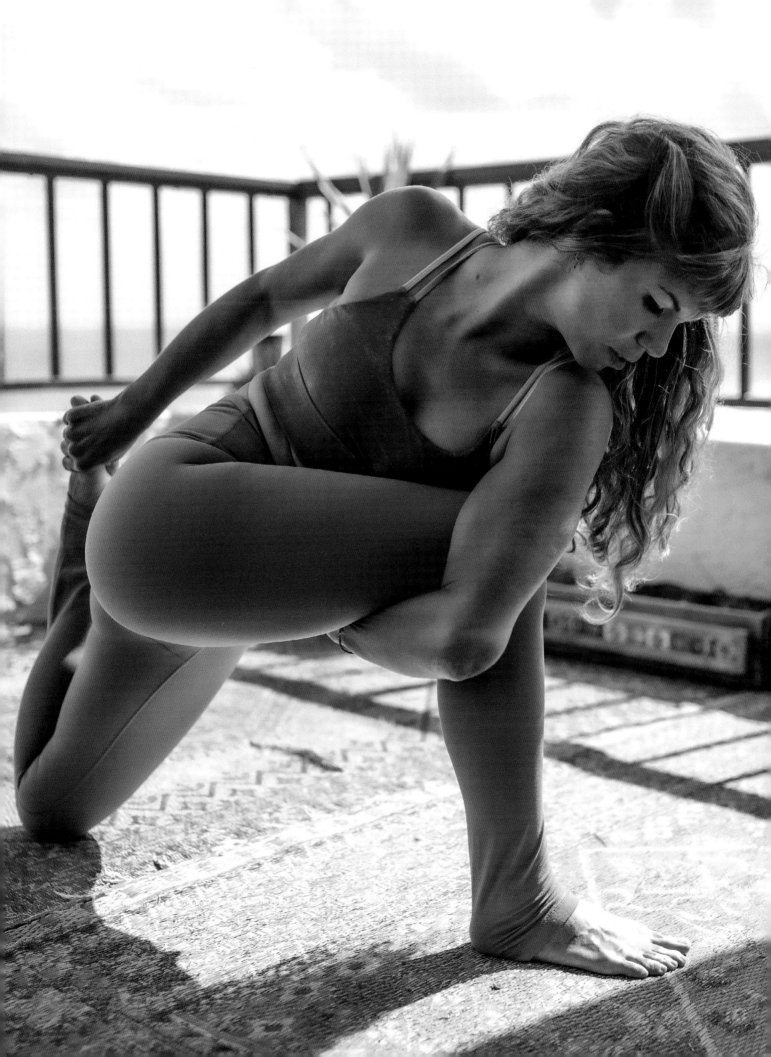

16. THEME: SAVOR

When we think of savoring something, we often think of a delicious meal or dessert, or perhaps a gorgeous sunset or sunrise, or a touching moment. But what if we also savored the transitions, the moments of change, our discomforts, and the challenges we face? When we arrive with the intention of savoring all of it, we can find that space where we can seek out whatever can be gleaned from any given moment rather than wishing it away. This mindfulness practice guides us to the awareness that the present moment (whether beautiful or hard to take) is the most important. Relishing, lingering, and therefore growing, and getting stronger and more flexible in body and mind—that's what we're here for. In other words, slowing down and savoring guides each and every one of us to be better. It's the journey of being our best selves!

In the early 2000s, when I was living in LA, I assisted Jerome Front on a silent yoga retreat at the Esalen Institute. I was the nanny for his two kids, and he was kind enough to give me this work-trade opportunity to experience the magic of Big Sur. Although we sat at communal tables, all of the meals were eaten in silence. The practice of silent meals was especially challenging because the food was delicious. We were meant to take the fork or spoon to our mouth for a bite, put the utensil down, fully chew what was in our mouth, then take the utensil for another bite and so on. It was truly remarkable how long it took to eat just a few bites of food when mindfully chewing each bite to its completion before taking the next. I sometimes say in jest that it was disappointing because often I couldn't finish my plate. Of course, eating more slowly and more mindfully, I was very tuned in to when I felt sated.

It was there in Big Sur where I learned the raisin meditation practice. Take a single raisin, look at it, all its grooves, the shine of it, the pattern of it. Then close your eyes to feel it, touch the stickiness of it, feel the squishiness of it. Bring it to your ear, listen to it as you rub it between your fingers, lightly squish it. Take the raisin to your nose and smell the sweetness. Then put it in your mouth without chewing it. Just feel it in your mouth, the grooves or crevices of the raisin against your tongue. And when you've explored all your senses with the raisin, then lightly start to chew this little raisin. Taste this burst of flavor on every taste bud you possess.

More often than not, most of us take handfuls of raisins to eat at a time and rush most of our meals. Perhaps it's not practical to savor every single moment, to make every bite so mindful. However, it's certainly something we can engage in more often than we think.

VIDEO: <u>Savor</u>

PLAYLIST: <u>Awake Me</u>

FEATURED SONG: <u>"Savor" by Matthew Mayer</u>

HIGHLIGHTED POSE/TRANSITION: Slow-motion evolution of Headstand.

JOURNAL PROMPT: *Choose one activity to savor this week. Maybe it's your morning coffee or tea, a meal, a conversation, an errand, a self-care routine, or time with a loved one.*

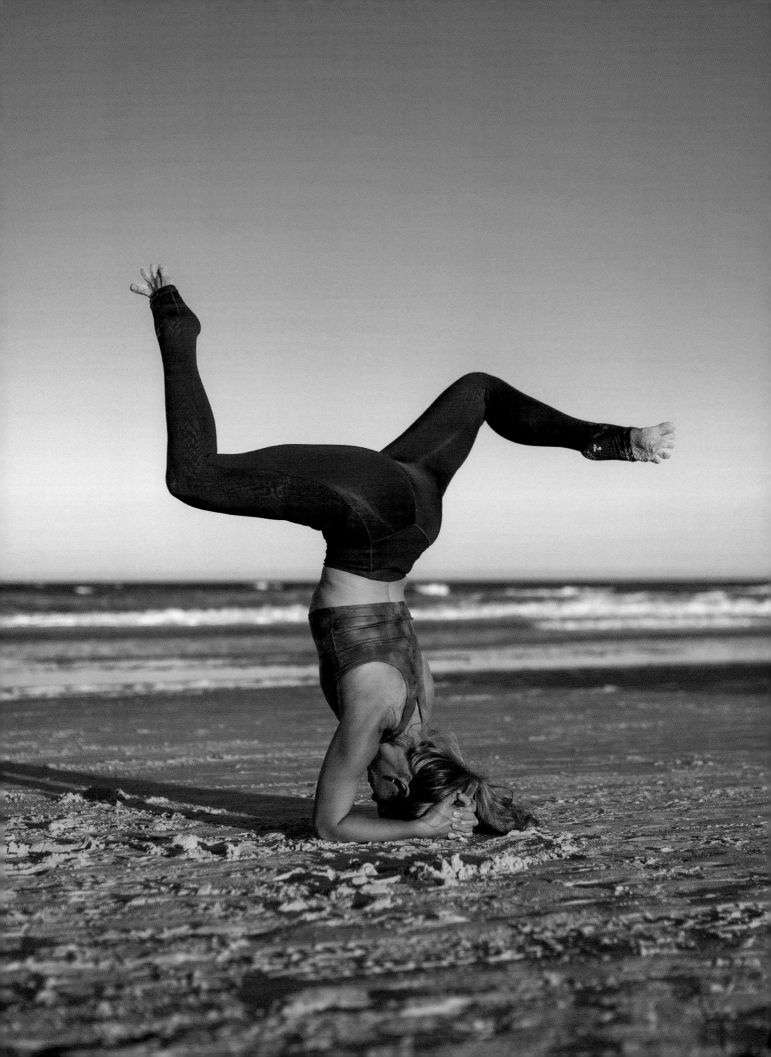

17. THEME: STAY CURIOUS

Embracing beginner's mind is one of my favorite practices for connecting with that childlike and playful quality within. When we arrive to each conversation from a space of curiosity, we have the ability to listen without bias. Take a look at all our habitual shapes in a yoga practice. Imagine you've never practiced downward-facing dog, for example. Close your eyes and feel this shape in your body, take a body scan, and linger here longer than you normally do. Where can you engage more? Where can you soften? This continuous evolution of self-observation can also be applied to the thoughts. Many of the thoughts we have are repeated. How curious! Contemplate why a story or thought continues to appear. This dive into the inner world will aid in freeing those thoughts that anchor you in the past or the future, and give you the awareness to guide yourself to the here and now.

In my twenties, I worked as a nanny for several families. Being around small children is one of the best ways to explore staying curious. I would love to take them outside to explore! A stick could become a magic wand, a rocket ship, a sword, a lollipop, a spoon for the most outlandish recipe… Imagination would run wild! We could be mixing the batter for a birthday cake and I'd ask, "What are we putting in the bowl?"

The kid would say, "Pickles!"

I'd say, "Pickles? In birthday cake?" They'd giggle. I'd play along, "Okay, what else?"

"Chocolate, gummy bears, syrup!"

"That sounds closer to a birthday cake," I'd say.

"Mud, spaghetti, goldfish crackers, and chicken nuggets," they'd say proudly.

"This sounds like a very interesting birthday cake," I'd say, miming tasting something undesirable. They'd laugh hysterically, rolling around on the ground. This "making of the cake" could go on for a while. In actuality, we were just sitting on the grass next to the jungle gym while I mimed stirring together the ingredients that they mimed throwing into the "bowl." But there was space to explore because we had no destination in mind. We truly could "embrace the journey," as the song goes.

It was great fun to see the world through the children's eyes. Their natural curiosity became infectious, and story-telling, creating music from found objects, making up songs about the moment, creating art with mixed mediums, and ultimately letting go of what makes sense, letting go of staying in the lines, and letting go of an agenda made all of my external stresses fade away.

VIDEO: <u>Stay Curious</u>

PLAYLIST: <u>Inspiration</u>

FEATURED SONG: <u>"Linger" by Freedom Fry</u>

HIGHLIGHTED POSE/TRANSITION: Exploration via cat-cow with intuitive and improvisational movement.

JOURNAL PROMPT: *Name just one thought that has been on repeat lately. Free write for five to ten minutes pondering why. Get it all out from a vantage point of nonjudgmental curiosity.*

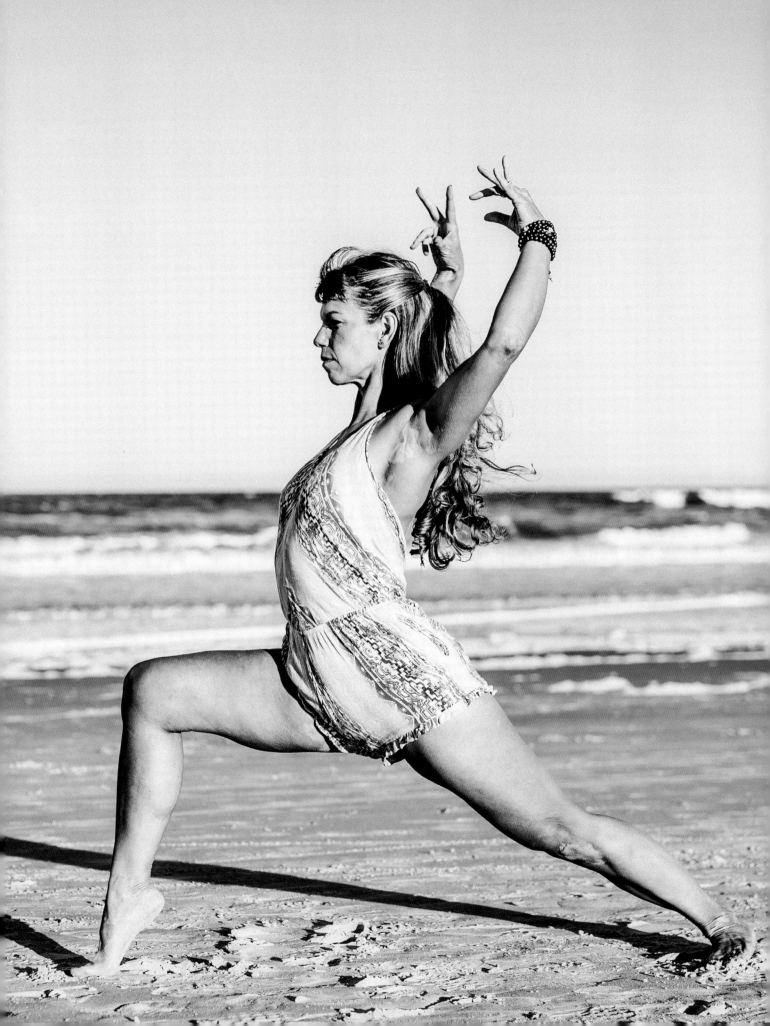

18. THEME: SOAK IN THE GOODNESS

Before soaking in the goodness, take a moment to observe the obstacles you have to surmount in order to embrace the goodness in you and in others. We'll embody the lotus flower, hold it to our hearts, and offer it up to the sky, first recognizing the beauty in ourselves as well as the beauty in others. The lotus is a gorgeous manifestation of the simple truth that, through the mud, beauty can emerge. And so can we. We can emerge through our suffering and fear and skepticism and resistance to change to carve out what may seem insignificant—a glimmer of goodness. The brain, as we know, is addicted to the thoughts we feed it, so why not feed it goodness? Soak it in and breathe into it. And breathe it out.

When I lived in NYC, I yearned to escape upstate as often as possible. As much as I loved the city, I felt at peace surrounded by trees. I actually felt like I could breathe more deeply. When leaving town wasn't possible, I began to practice finding my breath exactly where I was. On certain days, I would commit to really looking around me as I went from point A to point B. When living in an urban environment such as NYC, it can be easy to fall into the pattern of keeping your head in your phone or in a book, or listening to music or a podcast on the subway. I would sometimes play a game with myself: I'd try to notice if anyone simply was sitting on the train without doing something else. And don't get me wrong! I was often that person who was reading. I can't tell you how many times I missed my stop because I was so immersed in a book or a play. But during those times when I played that game with myself—one whole day to really take in all that was going on around me—I felt my soul was nourished. Nowhere else in the world can you hear such a multitude of languages on one train car, feeling the connection of so many different cultures and backgrounds, all bouncing along to our own respective destinations.

There was a time in my life when I felt like I was perpetually running five minutes late. I'd speed walk past all the tourists, focused only on getting where I was going as quickly as possible. When I allowed myself to slow down, I could take in a lot and relish the amazing buzz that came with living in such a vibrant city. On occasion, I'd stop and gaze at the Empire State Building. Just for a moment, I'd stand there, in the middle of the sidewalk, staring like a tourist. Those were some of my favorite moments. But, do you know, I lived there for nine years and never once went to the top?

Also among my favorite moments were those occasions when I got to see a phenomenal, life-changing, emotional play with my friend, Mateo. We'd walk wordlessly from the theatre, hand in hand, silently crying. I'd squeeze his hand and he'd squeeze mine. This knowing acknowledgment that we were changed somehow and had to quietly process this change, while a million other people walked past us on their own path, was something truly beautiful!

VIDEO: <u>Soak in the Goodness</u>

PLAYLIST: <u>Reflection</u>

FEATURED SONG: <u>"Patience" by The Lumineers</u>

HIGHLIGHTED POSES/TRANSITIONS: Lotus Mudra in easy seat, Crescent Lunge and Tree Pose.

JOURNAL PROMPT: *Discover a simple activity that feels like the perfect representation of goodness for you. Put in your calendar a recurring event of this feel-good goodness. This could be as often as you feel you can realistically commit to.*

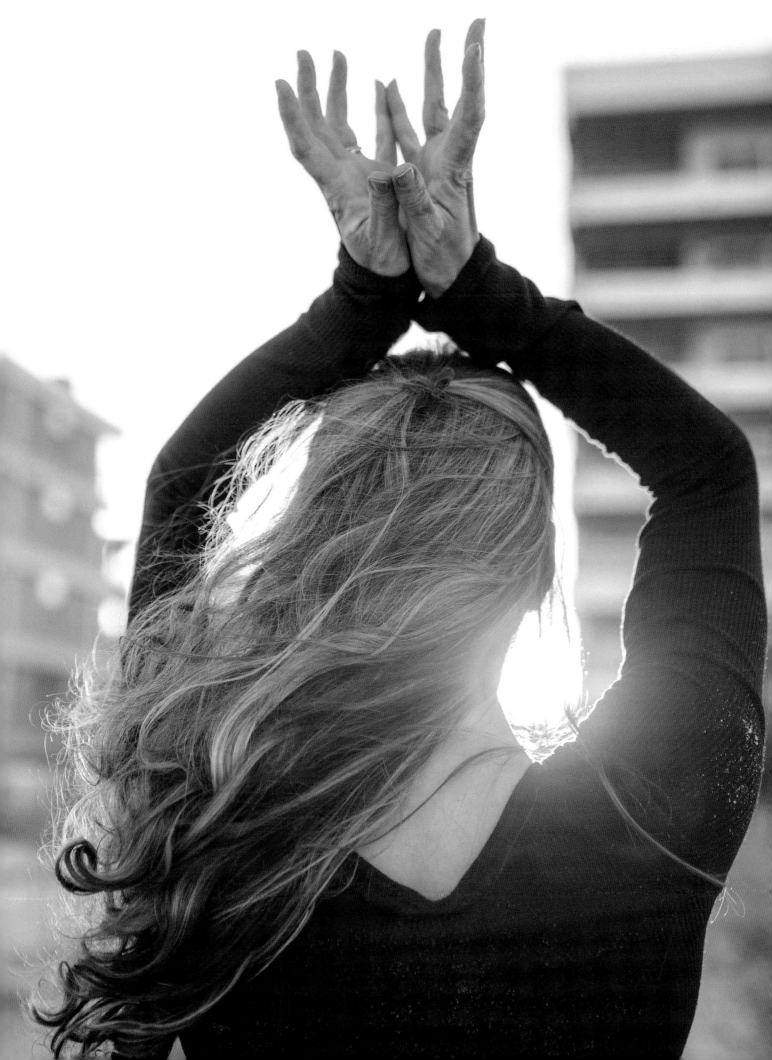

19. THEME: HEALING HABIT

Starting with a look at the asana yoga practice, notice if your modifications or your quest to embrace challenge are aiding your quest to heal, or impeding your body's restoration. Then turn inward and notice the thoughts surrounding past injuries. Guide your breath to a state of rest and restoration where your thoughts, words, and actions can all be united on your path to healing. There may be habits you have wanted to incorporate into your daily routine: a daily meditation practice, working on your balance, mindfulness during meals, or a home project you've been meaning to tackle for some time. Whatever it is, ask yourself where habit stacking (organizing similar tasks together) is possible. One of my new favorites is reading a spiritual passage while I'm waiting for the kettle to heat the water for my tea. It is just a few minutes, but it does set the tone for the day, and it helps guide me away from more time on my phone. Small healing habits each day add up over time. Begin with something easy to incorporate on a daily basis and breathe into the healing from within.

I've expanded my healing rituals considerably over the past year. What began as a quest to eat foods and beverages that are healing has developed into a fairly elaborate practice. I have now incorporated medicinal herbs and oils for the body and face, as well as a mindfulness surrounding all I do.

Or at least I try to.

What's funny is that I regarded myself as a pretty healthy person before my Ayurveda journey. I was vegetarian from age fourteen to age twenty-eight and vegan for the last two years. I mostly ate vegetables, but was less strict when I went out to eat. Zooming out and seeing myself from a distance, I recognize that while I exhibited some healthy habits, everything went out the window when I was busy, stressed, or busy and stressed all at once. I hadn't set a foundation for myself, particularly a morning ritual to ensure self-care was a top priority.

I'll be honest and share that I still struggle with this sometimes. Though I intend to have a beautiful salad for lunch, sometimes that becomes a macrobar in my car between clients. Part of the practice is being aware, taking the time to carve space for one healing habit at a time, and of course having compassion for yourself when you falter. We all falter sometimes. Take a breath and begin again.

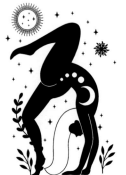

VIDEO: <u>Healing Habit</u>

PLAYLIST: <u>You Can't Rush Your Healing</u>

FEATURED SONG: <u>"Spirit Bird" by Xavier Rudd</u>

HIGHLIGHTED POSES/TRANSITIONS: Cow face legs with prayer twist, unwind into forward fold with option to invert into headstand with eagle legs.

JOURNAL PROMPT: *Name one healing habit you're ready to incorporate to your weekly or daily routine.*

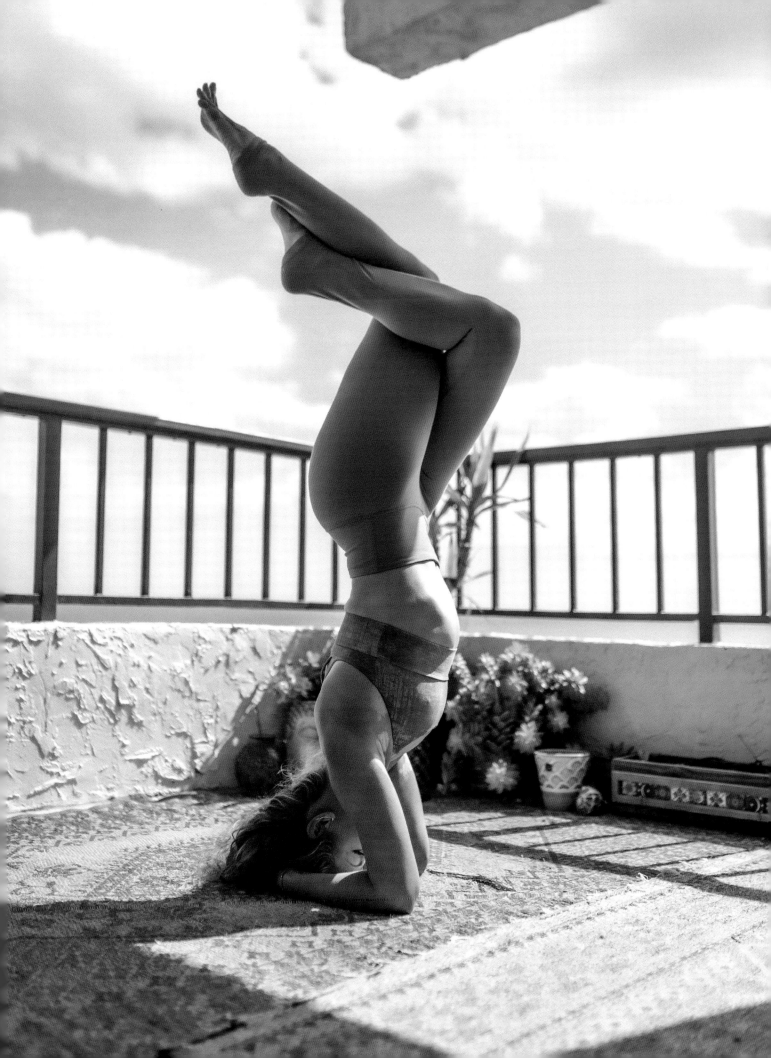

20. THEME: BE ALIGNED

We observe the alignment in each shape, linking breath to movement, while also tuning inward. How do your thoughts influence your words, and how do your words manifest in your actions? They could manifest as self-doubt for a particular pose, or perhaps self-doubt in the way you're living your life. So today, take a moment to check in with your edge in the yoga practice on the mat. Notice if your mind is convincing you that you are or aren't capable of something and simply give it a try. As we continue to show up and shift our awareness of what we previously believed was possible in our yoga practice, we can then embody more possibilities off the mat as well. Play with shifting from fear to seeking inspiration and notice how this shift in mindset can aid in aligning you with a life inspired.

If you've ever been to LA, you've likely remarked that everywhere you can eavesdrop you will hear a conversation about the entertainment industry. Almost everyone around you is a writer, actor, director, producer, or an aspiring one of the aforementioned. When I first arrived in LA, I took what everyone said at face value. Over the years, I came to understand that many people talk about making movies; however, very few actually do. And it's not just about whether someone follows through with the film they've been talking about writing for ten years. If what they are saying is out of alignment from what they are doing in this aspect, chances are they are misaligned overall.

Do your thoughts translate to your words, and do your words translate to your actions? Do you feel like you are in alignment with a version of yourself that vibrates, illuminates, and radiates? If there is a disconnect here, look inward. Trace your thoughts down the portal to their source. When did you first start thinking this? When did you first begin believing this? Is this your truth, or were you convinced of it by external sources? What if what you think isn't true? Does this change what you say? Does this shift what you do? Does this change feel liberating, scary, uncomfortable, untethered?

Close your eyes and see the version of yourself that vibrates, illuminates, and radiates. What does this version of yourself think? What does this version of yourself say? And what does this version of yourself do? You have the power to reprogram the thought patterns in your head. For example, if you are feeling overwhelmed and stressed out, the thought might be, "Ugh, I'll never be able to complete everything on time." Then, you might say, "I'm going to be late." And, voila! You manifest yourself as late. Take the same circumstance and try this. Think, "Inhale, I'm completing this one most important task today." Then say, "It feels so gratifying to complete the most important thing." And voila! You manifest yourself as calm, collected, and in control of what is most important. Of course I'm simplifying for the sake of the example, but take from it whatever you find helpful.

VIDEO: <u>Be Aligned</u>

PLAYLIST: <u>Be the Change</u>

FEATURED SONG: <u>"I Release Control" by Alexa Sunshine Rose</u>

HIGHLIGHTED POSES/TRANSITIONS: Open hip shapes with attention to knee alignment, building to flying pigeon.

JOURNAL PROMPT: *Write down a mantra that inspires you. Repeat it whenever you find you are straying away from your alignment with your highest intentions.*

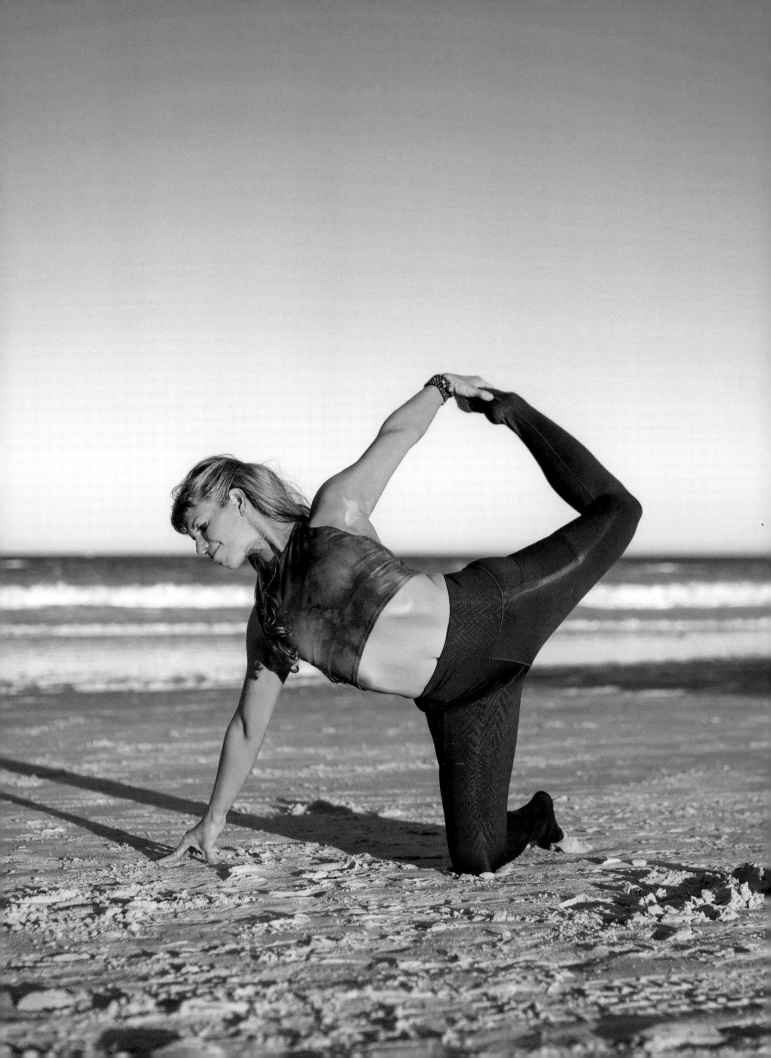

21. THEME: SHIFT PERSPECTIVE

First, discover an awareness of your thoughts and your knee-jerk response to challenge, change, or something unexpected. How can we change the lens through which we view the world, almost like trying on funky sunglasses with different tints? Very often in the past year, I have heard and read about people getting fed up with 2020 and wishing it away. While such sentiments are understandable, rather than wishing the year would end, how might we shift to see what can be gleaned from this time—what can be learned—and how we might utilize this time to strengthen and grow?

This is not to block off heartache, frustration, resentment, grief, or fear. But, rather, observe when limiting emotions are lingering in the driver's seat for too long. The same person who says, "I can't do yoga because I'm not strong or flexible enough," might say, "I can't do 2020 because it's too challenging." They very well may be right in their own self-fulfilling prophecy. But what if we empower ourselves to change the narrative? "I breathe into what is, and trust that all I need is already within me."

Sometimes, when mulling over a decision, I will literally shift my perspective: performing a headstand or a handstand, or just lying on my back with my legs thrown over the couch. If I'm inside, I might go outside to take my dog to the park or go to the beach. Sometimes switching up your routine can provide you with a new point of view. If you have the ability to take your work outside, take your work outside! The sun and the fresh air can certainly aid in productivity and help you feel inspired. If you tend to sit down most of the day, I invite you to set a timer to remind you to stand up, stretch your legs, do some stretches, or walk around the block every thirty minutes or so. Alternately, if you're on your feet most of the day, I invite you to sit down with a tall spine, take some stretches, and come into your breath.

One of my favorite activities to bring joy into my entire mind, body, and soul is to host my own private dance party in the kitchen. I put on Spotify's fun morning songs playlist and I dance without inhibition. I turn the music up really loud and rock out to my heart's content. Sometimes I arrive to my own dance party a little reluctant, but finding choice music is key to letting the body move. It is therapeutic to shake up the entire system, stimulate the blood flow, let the music take you, and let go.

VIDEO: <u>Shift Perspective</u>

PLAYLIST: <u>Rest Assured</u>

FEATURED SONG: <u>"Fix Me Up" by Ayo</u>

HIGHLIGHTED POSES/TRANSITIONS: Headstand with ankles crossed or legs up the wall. Yin practice of shapes typically upright taken on the back, such as the reclined sleeping swan.

JOURNAL PROMPT: *Describe a recent time when you overcame a challenge by shifting the way you perceived the situation.*

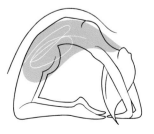

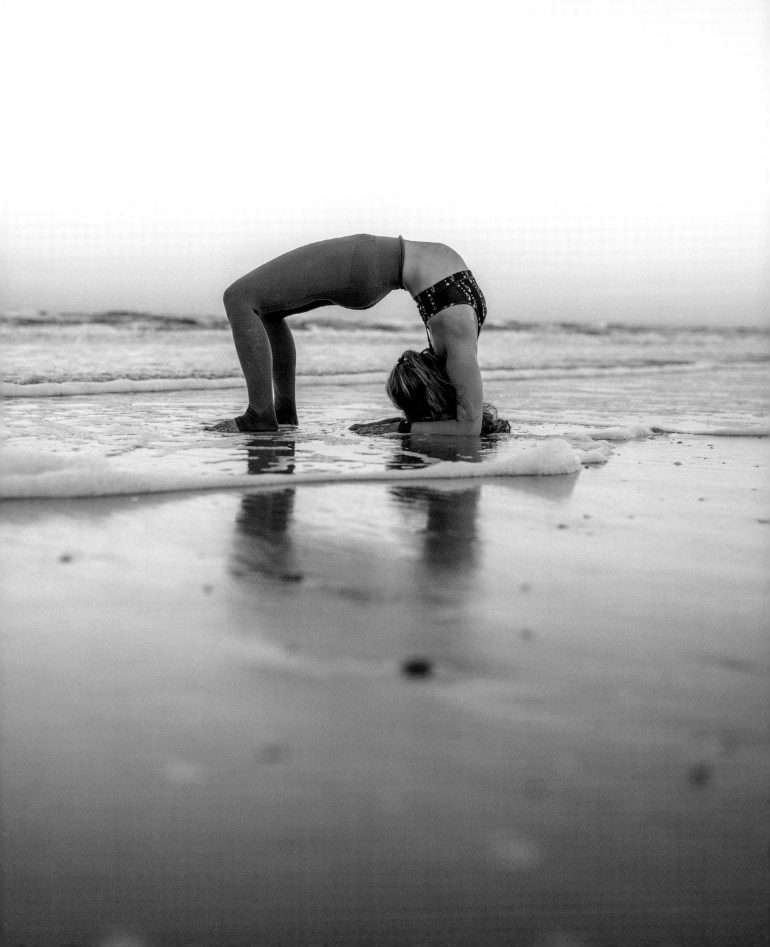

22. THEME: STAY AWAKE

Awaken to the present moment with newfound inspiration. We will move our bodies and come to our edge of discomfort as a way to discover something new in the habitual. As we continue to be tempted to shut down and go back to sleep, perhaps the greatest discoveries can be made when we breathe through the discomfort a little bit longer. We can awaken to a new purpose with new excitement. Dust off the cobwebs of old dreams and perhaps let go of old ambitions that no longer ring true. Greet this day with awe, rub your eyes, and take a giant stretch. Embrace this fresh canvas before you!

My friend Stacey jokingly dubbed the ongoing days of lockdowns and quarantines as "Blursday," because they all seem to sort of blur together. I often find myself recounting a story, saying things like, "On Thursday—wait, I think it was Wednesday—last week. Or was it Friday? Ha, one day last week." When we are immersed in routine, we sometimes revert to autopilot and the days do indeed blur together. When I catch myself almost checking out, I make it a point to wake up earlier the next day.

Trust me, I am not a morning person. I never have been, even as a kid. My parents will attest to this. In this new chapter of my life, however, I have enjoyed awakening with the sunrise or slightly beforehand. Following my morning beverages, journaling, and reading, I like to pull out my bullet journal with my calendar. I write down all the things that must be done, including appointments. I write some things that I would like to get done, and others that might be more back-burner things. Something about taking pen to paper and getting all of that out of my head is liberating to me. It's the first step to actually completing the tasks. Ideally, I've also carved enough time to move my body in some way before I do anything else. This is transformative to me! And all before turning my phone back on from the night before! This is how I stay tuned in to what's going on with my body, what's going on with my mind. I regard this morning ritual as the safeguarding of my soul against anything that can come my way during the day. It's the way I stay present.

VIDEO: <u>Stay Awake</u>

PLAYLIST: <u>Let Go</u>

FEATURED SONG: <u>"I Won't Give Up" by Jason Mraz</u>

HIGHLIGHTED POSES/TRANSITIONS: Fire toe pose, movement in cat-cow into downward-facing dog.

JOURNAL PROMPT: *What is your favorite way to naturally awaken both your mind and body?*

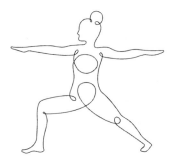

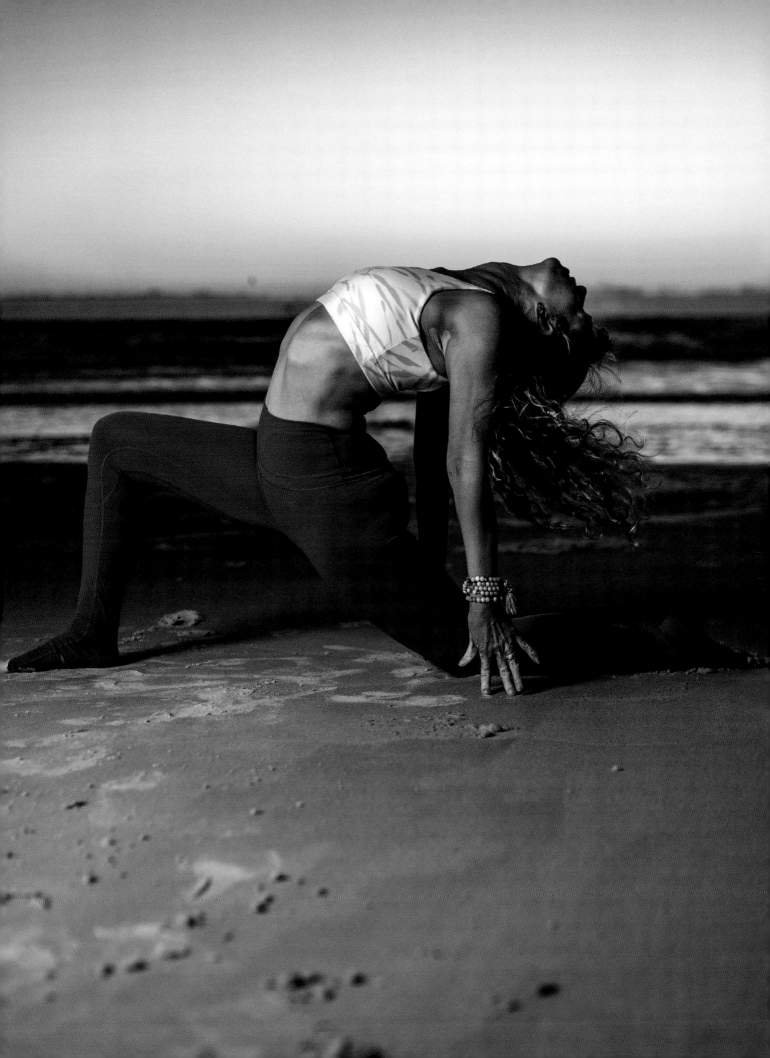

23. THEME: TAKE REST

If you're anything like me, you tend to take rest only when you're ill, you have an injury, or some other major life change forces rest upon you. It is both my hope and my intention to practice in the spirit of a marathon rather than a sprint, so that I can continue to practice all of my days. But I also try to remember that sometimes a complete day of rest is in order. I remind myself that on occasion it's alright to practice at 30–70 percent of your ability. While I love a good to-do list, enjoy being productive, and excel at multitasking, the fact is, I'm called to do less these days in order to preserve my energy, and I invite you to do the same. We cannot pour from an empty cup, so conserving our energy is not only important as a self-care practice but also to ensure we can be available to our loved ones.

Part of taking rest means saying no sometimes. And, oh my, saying no is hard for me! At the beginning of the year, I was teaching every day and at almost every yoga studio or wellness center in town. When the studios all closed due to COVID, I decided to start carving space for myself to rest. I struggled with letting go of most of my classes because my heart felt tethered to each class in a different way. I knew deep down that if I gave myself the space, I could feel more inspired to create new inventive sequencing and cultivate themes that resonate both with me and with my students.

Somehow, some way, I currently have one and sometimes even two days off a week. Do I plan classes, work on marketing, and take care of administrative tasks on these days? You know I do. Taking rest is hard for me. However, I am trying to take breaks as often as I can manage to tear myself away from my to-do list. When I catch myself, I take my dog for a walk or catch up with a friend in person or on the phone. For some, rest looks something like sitting down with a good book, while for others, rest looks something like going on a brisk walk along the beach. Sometimes it depends on whether stillness or movement feels more therapeutic in the moment.

VIDEO: <u>Take Rest</u>

PLAYLIST: <u>Mellow Friday</u>

FEATURED SONG: <u>"The Only Thing" by Sufjan Stevens</u>

HIGHLIGHTED POSES/TRANSITIONS: Find ease in flow and in stillness.
Lie down on your back with fingers interlaced behind your head. Close your
eyes and begin to star gaze or cloud watch in your mind's eye.

JOURNAL PROMPT: *What restful activity will you incorporate into your routine this week?*

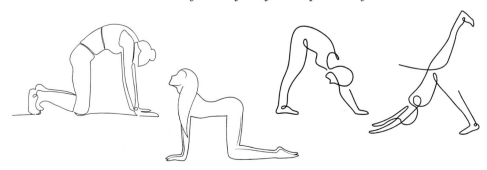

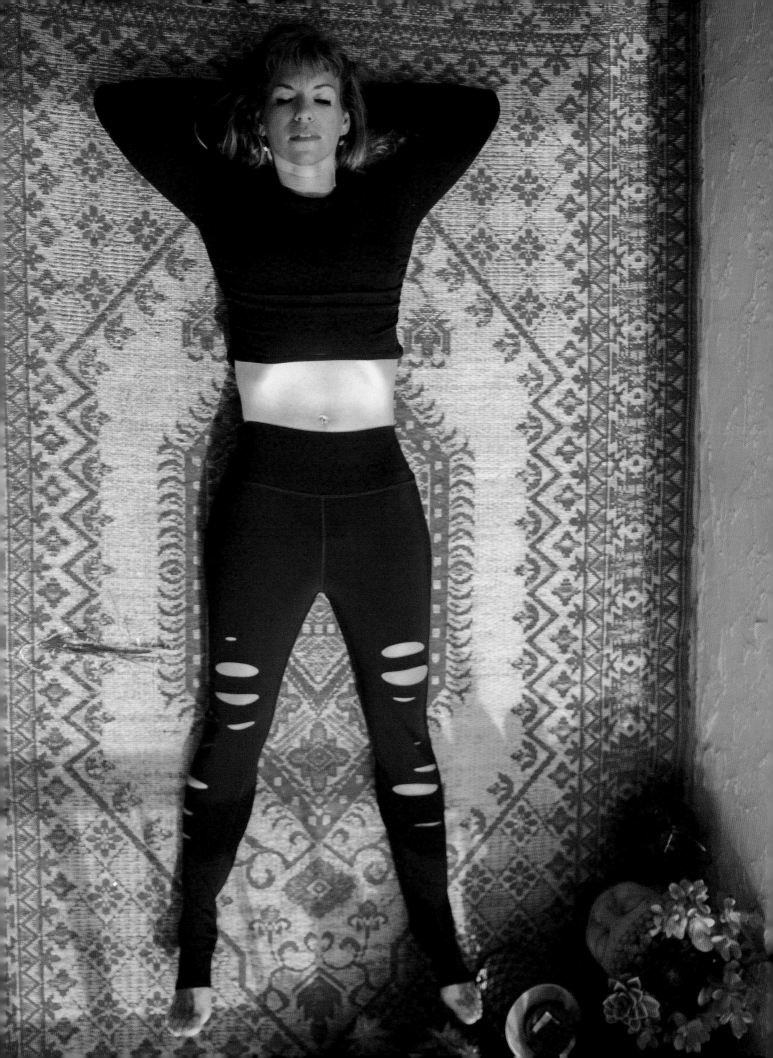

24. THEME: COOL AND SOOTHE

Whether practicing Yin or Yang styles of asana yoga, we can experience heat within. Maybe your heat within lives there always, or maybe you experience heat with rising emotions, or overheat with physical exertion. Regardless, we can all benefit from practicing cooling breath as we guide our thoughts to self-soothe.

In the dog days of summer, the mind will do its best to convince you that you will be calm once the temperature cools down. The temperature of our body and our temperament are often connected. When we are hot, we tend to get irritable, agitated, angry, fearful. So if we can guide ourselves to arrive to situations with a cool and soothing feel and mindset, we become adept at allowing conflict to roll off our backs with more grace and ease. Finding coolness within also breaks the mindset of "When _____ happens, then I'll be calm, peaceful, happy." Empower yourself to feel, breathe, and believe that even when it's 100 degrees outside, you can find a sense of cooling and soothing sensation within.

One of the attributes I inherited from my father's side is I run HOT! Or I suppose I should say I used to run hot. I was that person in the middle of winter standing on the subway in just a tank top, my many shed layers draped over my arm. I would of course wear my "sleeping bag" coat to go outside, but whenever I arrived at my location, I would instantly start taking off layers. It's funny to see photos of past gatherings where everyone around me is wearing sweaters, sometimes even hats and scarves, and there I am in a tank top.

As I mentioned previously, before my Ayurveda journey, I was a HUGE coffee drinker. I loved, loved, LOVED my morning coffee ritual, and I often would put my coffee in a thermos to carry with me from class to class, sipping from it throughout the day. I could even have coffee after dinner and experience no difficulties going to sleep. I used to joke that "coffee just brings me into balance." I never felt jittery or suffered any negative effects. So when my Ayurveda consultant suggested I quit coffee, I truly was resistant. It was the first thing I did in the morning, before anything else.

When I began my Ayurveda journey, I was interested in cooling my system, especially now that I live in Florida. What I love about this practice—or one of the things I love about it—is its focus on bringing the body back into balance. Once a certain equilibrium is established, we can respond to outside stimulus with more grace.

I have now incorporated several herbs and rituals into my daily routine that cool and soothe my entire system. One of my favorite practices is having a large glass of water with a squeeze of lime first thing in the morning, before any other beverage. It helps cleanse and reset my system before I introduce tea (not coffee) or anything else.

VIDEO: Cool and Soothe

PLAYLIST: Hold On, Again

FEATURED SONG: "Inner Peace" by Beautiful Chorus

HIGHLIGHTED POSE/TRANSITION: Cooling pranayama.

JOURNAL PROMPT: *Name three actions you can take to cool yourself down when you are overheated physically or emotionally.*

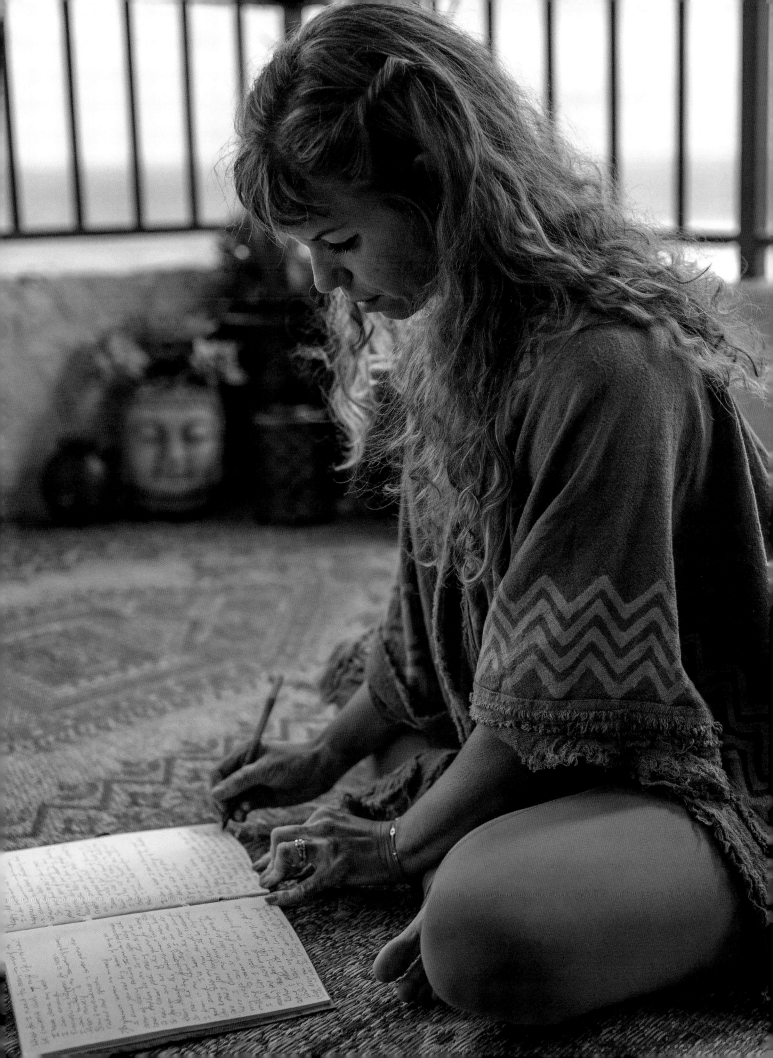

25. THEME: YOU ALREADY DO

The secret to having it all is knowing you already do. Breathe this in. Breathe this out. Shift your awareness from what once was or what may be to what is. Let go of the tangibles that lure you into thinking "I need that" when confronted with those things (relationships, status, etc.) you don't have that you believe will complete you. The more you breathe into acceptance of all you already possess, the more you can embody this mindfulness and meditation practice in all you do.

To all my fellow type As out there, this is a hard concept to make peace with. Does this mean we should throw our hands up and stop striving for more? I don't believe so. Does this mean we must let go of our dreams of the idyllic home, or of select tangible items on our wish lists? Probably not. The point is how we approach our priorities, making sure to take the time to delight in all we already have.

When I practice gratitude, you know I'm breathing in thankfulness for having a roof over my head, a very comfy bed, shoes to protect my feet, and a variety of clothes to express the way I feel. If we lived in this home with these tangible items for the rest of our days, would it be enough? Of course it would. And yet I hope to move one day, in the next few years, to my dream home. It's funny, right?

I said to my mom the other day, "Do you think there will ever be a point where we stop with all the home projects or the striving for more things to buy?"

She stopped for a moment to ponder this and then finally replied, "I think there will always be something."

So how do we balance our drive with our contentment? I think it shows up in the everyday. Are you working so hard that you're missing seeing your loved ones? Or are you already in your dream home, but so consumed with all that needs to be done, you're missing the part where you enjoy the gorgeous pool in the backyard?

In modern times, it can feel challenging to stop, appreciate the view, and sit down solely for the purpose of sitting, breathing, and expressing gratitude for all we already have. The acknowledgment that what you have is enough is the bridge to a lasting joy.

VIDEOS: <u>You Already Do</u>

PLAYLIST: <u>Reflection</u>

FEATURED SONG: <u>"Patience" by The Lumineers</u>

HIGHLIGHTED POSES/TRANSITIONS: Happy baby and forward folds.

JOURNAL PROMPT: *What do I need to be happy, content in a fulfilling way? Write down the things you need versus the things you want. Then notice if you can embody the things you need or want to be happy in the here and now. We can strive for more while accepting where we are in the present. And knowing this is enough.*

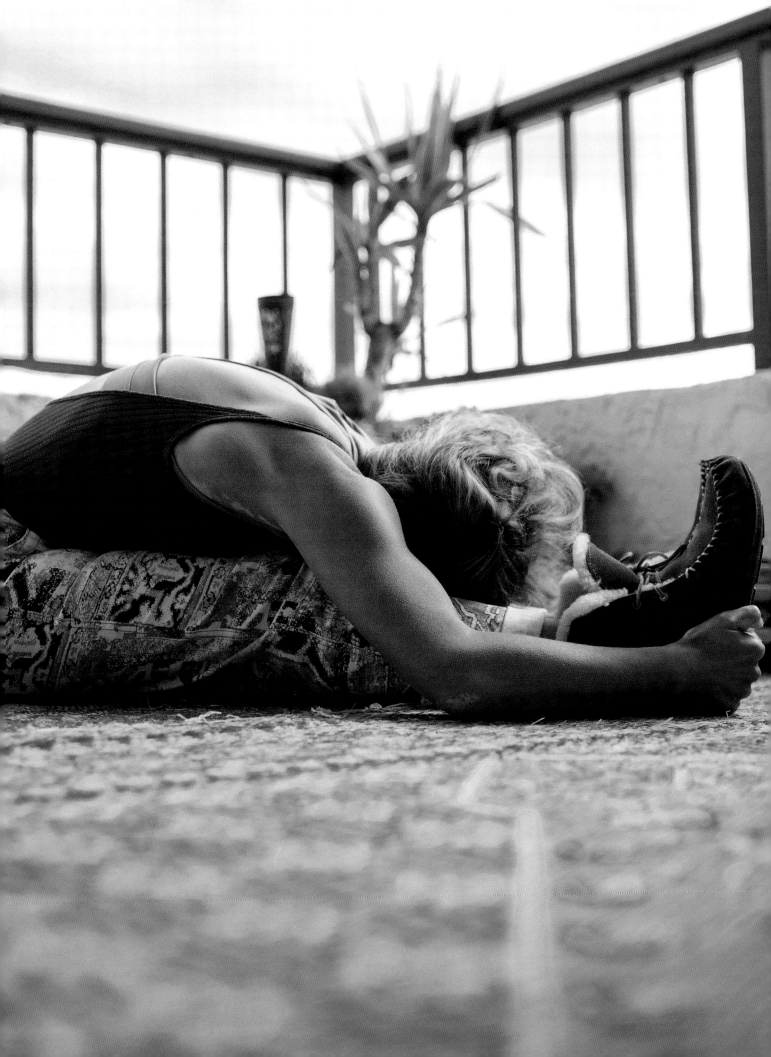

26. THEME: UNPLUG & UNWIND

Now more than ever, we can connect directly with people from all over the world. We have information at our fingertips and an abundance of distractions literally in the palm of our hands. The world has opened itself up to us with the speed of the Internet, and all those bright lights and moving images have taken us out of the present moment. Just for today, or maybe for the whole week, play with turning your phone off at night and leaving it off for ten to sixty minutes (or even longer!) after you wake up. Turn off "push notifications" on your social media. If you are in the middle of something and the phone rings or sounds a text alert, resist looking at it immediately. Finish what you are doing and then mindfully look when you are ready and when you can thoughtfully respond. Most things don't require an urgent response. Turn the TV or music off when you're eating and try not to look at your phone during your meals. When we eat mindfully, the food tastes better and we realize we are full sooner. These are suggestions to unplug and unwind off the mat.

On the mat, notice if there is an invisible tether from your brain to something that happened earlier or that might happen later. Try to breathe into letting go or unplugging from these low-energy habits and guide yourself to vibrate higher with inspired creativity, vibrant breath, and sustained focus on the here and now.

When I was in Costa Rica doing my first yoga teacher training with Amazing Yoga, I stayed in a tent. There were a lot of stairs from the tents to where we would practice and I was hot most of the time. I was simultaneously remotely recasting a play I was both producing and acting in with my theatre company and fielding a lot of drama coming at me from New York. I was pretty much an emotional wreck. It felt like everything about the life I was building was against me, even though I poured every ounce of my energy into it! I didn't truly believe it at the time, but my yoga teacher training was the beginning of me letting go of my theatre company, and the beginning of me letting go of my pursuits as an actor. I had hit my head against the brick wall many times and for many years!

I stayed in Costa Rica for another week following my yoga teacher training for a yoga retreat with Cortney Ostrosky. My mom came to join me. The last night of the retreat there was a fire ceremony. We all wrote something on a piece of paper and then threw it in the fire as an expression of truly letting it go. I wrote, "That I must suffer for my art." Somehow along the way I had come to believe I must starve, be miserable, and carry tons of anxiety in pursuit of my craft. This was all very deeply buried, however. On the surface, for the most part, I was living my dream, meeting amazing and inspiring collaborators, and building my legacy.

This time in Costa Rica was the first step on my journey from merely surviving to actually thriving. It would be another two or three years before I fully let go, but, oh my goodness, I'm so grateful I did!

VIDEO: <u>Unplug and Unwind</u>
PLAYLIST: <u>Let Go</u>
FEATURED SONG: <u>"Let It All Go"</u> by Birdy, RHODES

HIGHLIGHTED POSES/TRANSITIONS: Twisted chair pose and child's pose.

JOURNAL PROMPT: *What are you ready to let go of? What's one thing you can do today to prepare yourself to let go?*

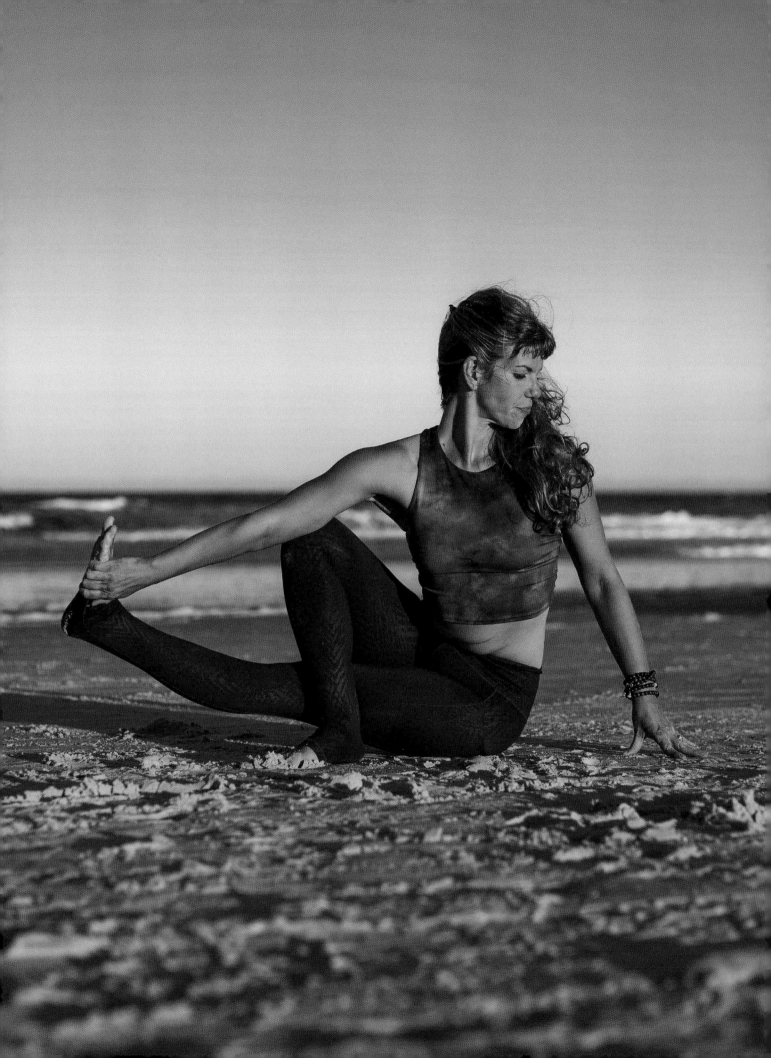

27. THEME: CONNECTION

Surround yourself with people whose eyes light up when they see you coming.

—*Andre de Shields*

In this time of social distancing, I have come to miss many things about sharing space with others: giving and receiving hands-on assists in yoga class, being mat to mat in rooms full of people united by the desire to be the best version of themselves, breathing into the now and exhaling loudly through the mouth. We've now spent six months six feet apart and the separation is palpable when I try to smile at someone through my mask. But this physical separation is out of my control. It's out of all of our control! So how can we find peace with this new normal?

We can connect beginning from within. We can connect mind and body. We can connect breath per movement. We can connect grounding into the earth and lifting up to the sky. And we can use sense memory to feel a loving assist of the shoulders or the hips.

Until we can safely hug and gather without fear, this visualization of connection, making the most of those things we do have control over, is surprisingly calming. We can take this deep-seated connection with us out into the world. We can make eye contact and say hello to those we see and seek out the smile from behind the mask that reveals itself in the eyes. And we can FaceTime with loved ones we miss just because, or pick up the phone and check in on everyone who touches our heart as a way to touch theirs. We can stay connected in this way—in our thoughts, in our breath, in our words, and in our actions.

My favorite connection practices these days are practicing yoga with Bowery by my side, weekly tennis drills, shopping excursions or spa days with my mom, and weekly walks with my friend Stacey, where we talk about all things sans edit button and get to feel this cathartic release in both mind and body.

VIDEO: <u>Connection</u>

PLAYLIST: <u>Reflection</u>

FEATURED SONG: <u>"Light Years" by The National</u>

HIGHLIGHTED POSES/TRANSITIONS: **Moving breath per movement, movement within shapes, and then flowing.**

JOURNAL PROMPT: *List five ways you'll connect with yourself and others this week.*

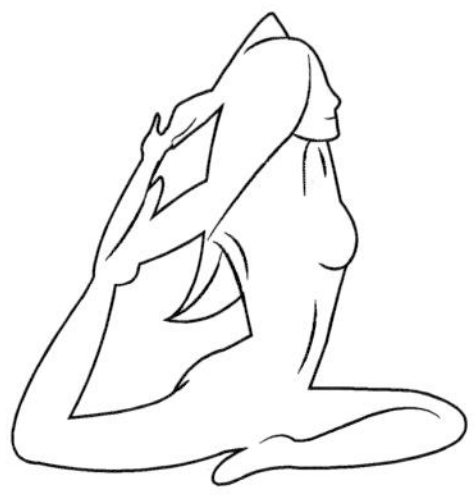

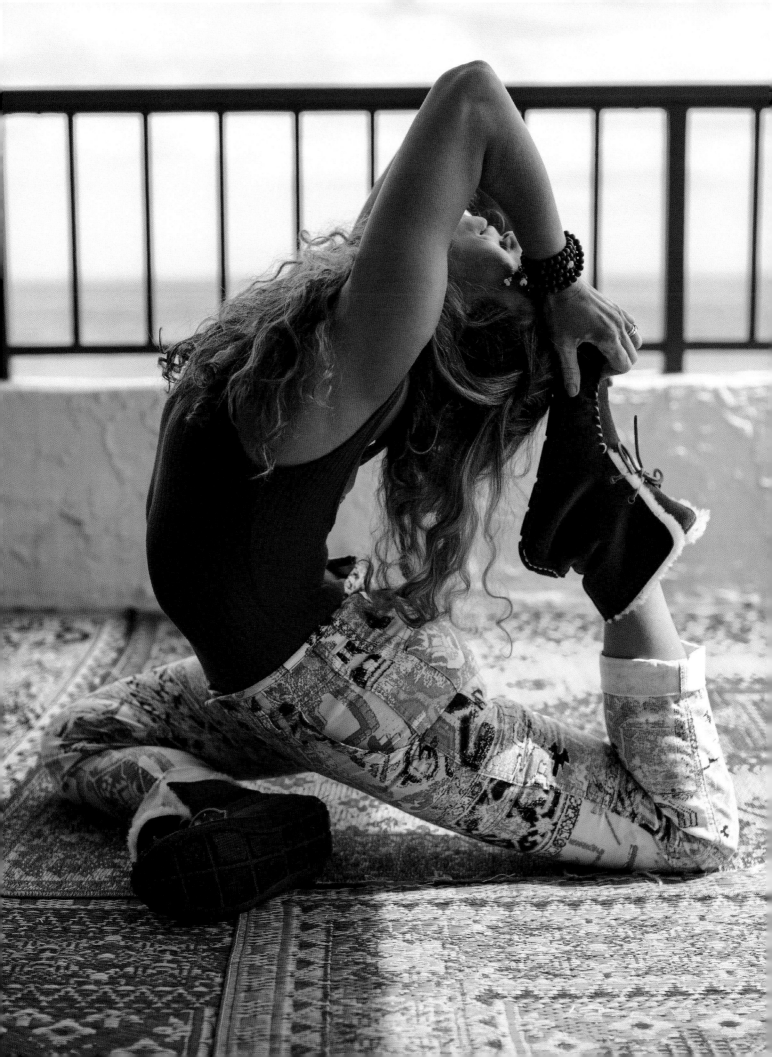

28. THEME: UNTANGLE YOUR HEART

Whether deeply buried or close to the surface, we all have cracks, breaks, tears, or knots in our hearts. These emotional wounds may come from past or current relationships, from messy encounters, from our own thoughts that have amplified situations, or simply from being alive. What would it mean to untangle one of these knots? If you feel ready, explore letting go of a tangle holding you back from living your best life and fully immersing yourself into all you can be.

We'll explore breathing into the heart space, breathing healing energy with intention. We're exploring shapes where we expose the heart to breathe into both the strength and the vulnerability that resides there and, in our forward folds, breathing into the back of the heart, filling up the hidden crevices. As we open up the heart space physically, it really does transform the way we breathe, which has a direct impact on our thoughts and emotional lives. When we crack our hearts open in this beautiful gesture of "I'm ready, I'm open, I'm here!" we can see our way out of the tangles anew.

In my physical practice, I adore all the heart openers! I also happen to have a lot of mobility in my spine and shoulders so these shapes come fairly easily to me. I think the emotional aspect of these shapes deeply resonates with me as well. I regard myself as someone who loves with every cell of my being. So I feel this quite profoundly in my asana practice, my heart exclaiming, "I'm here for you!"

For many years as both a student and a teacher, I would set the intention at the beginning of class as simply "Love." It represented a love for the teacher and the teachers before us, a love for the yoga practice and all of its teachings, a love for my body just as it is—moving my being through space and expressing shapes that light me up and inspire me—a love for the community around me, and a love of the beautiful practice of breathing together, moving together, and creating space for each of our respective lights to shine brightly.

VIDEO: <u>Untangle Your Heart</u>

PLAYLIST: <u>Humble Me</u>

FEATURED SONG: <u>"Forgive" by Trevor Hall, Luka Lesson</u>

HIGHLIGHTED POSE/TRANSITION: Humble Warrior, crack your heart open to prepare.

JOURNAL PROMPT: *How can you open your heart to others this week?*

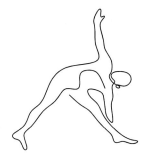

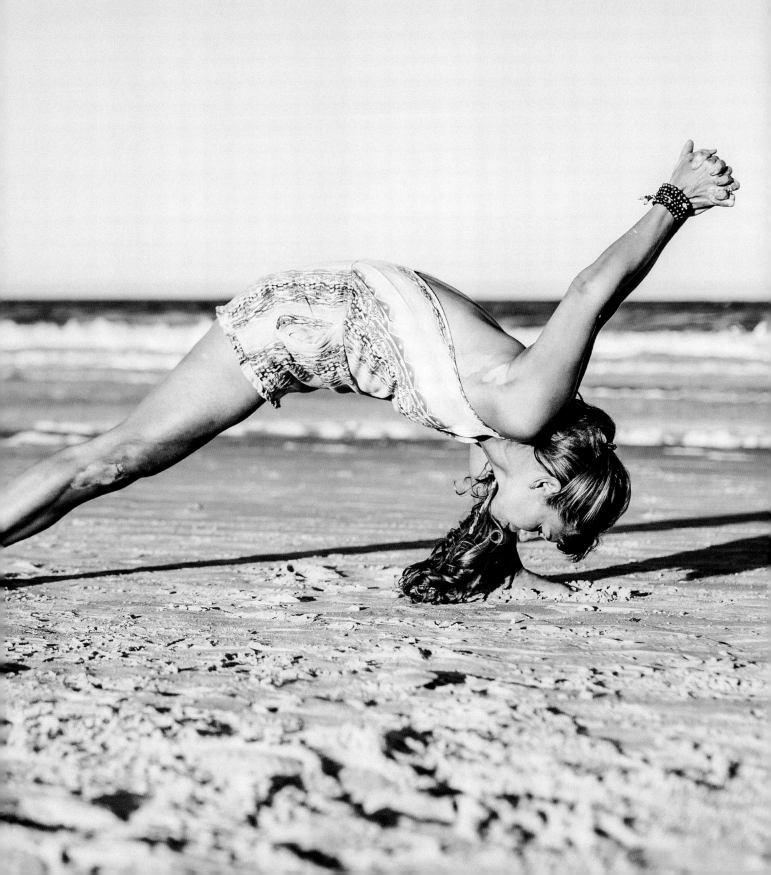

29. THEME: GROUNDING

What does grounding mean to you? And what quality would you need to possess in order to feel grounded, however that word resonates with you? Observe yourself on the earth; feel that tether and that rootedness. One of my favorite parts of embodying trees in the yoga practice is the reminder to feel the earth, to breathe and move with the winds and feel uplifted with growth. Visualize the part of your body and your clothing making contact with your yoga mat, the floor, the carpet, or the earth directly. Allow this visualization to become a beautiful watercolor painting so that the colors of your clothes and skin blend with the colors of your mat, the floor, the earth. As we begin to delineate less between where our body begins and ends and where the earth begins and ends, we can feel more connected and more at peace.

I recently was guided through an empathy introspection meditation by Sean Imler as part of my five-hundred-hour advanced yoga teacher training with Authentic Movements. He's brilliant and provides intelligent guidance into the mindfulness practice. In this introspection, I was able to feel unbelievably grounded by his visualization cues. This reinforced the power of meditation, introspection, and visualization—the overarching power of our minds. Ultimately, nothing had "changed" from before the meditation to after the meditation and yet somehow it had. The external circumstances remain and yet my inner world is transformed.

As we continue to delve more into learning about ourselves—what triggers us, what lights us up, what destroys our spirit, what annoys us, what excites us, what sends us reeling into harmful habits, and what anchors us—we can better navigate how to discover and rediscover balance in our mind, body, and soul.

One of my favorite grounding practices, one that often serves as inspiration for journaling, is taking walks outside. This could be just around the neighborhood, or discovering a new path somewhere, or going to the beach. But I have plenty of others! I also love being in water—the pool, the ocean, a bath, a hot tub—it doesn't matter. If you're a water baby like me, I hope you find water often. Even looking at water feels amazingly grounding to me. You know by now I'm all about journaling! Every morning I do a short journaling practice in the five-year spiritual journal my friend Leah gave me. It's grounding to know I will do that every morning, answering a prompt and also reading what I've written in the past couple of years. And of course, you know I have to say my yoga practice! Sometimes that looks like a guided meditation, breathing practice, moving my body organically or through guidance (whether alone or in a group), eating without distraction, taking a breath when I feel triggered, practicing gratitude, mantra or mala meditation, studying yoga history and philosophy, or simply pausing sometimes to feel my feet on the earth and acknowledge all the abundance I possess.

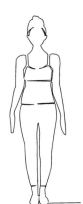

VIDEO: <u>Grounding</u>

PLAYLIST: <u>Awake Me</u>

FEATURED SONG: <u>"Savor" by Matthew Mayer</u>

HIGHLIGHTED POSES/TRANSITIONS: Mountain Pose, Warrior I and Warrior III, and Tree Pose on our backs, and finding these shapes standing.

JOURNAL PROMPT: *What does grounding mean to you?*

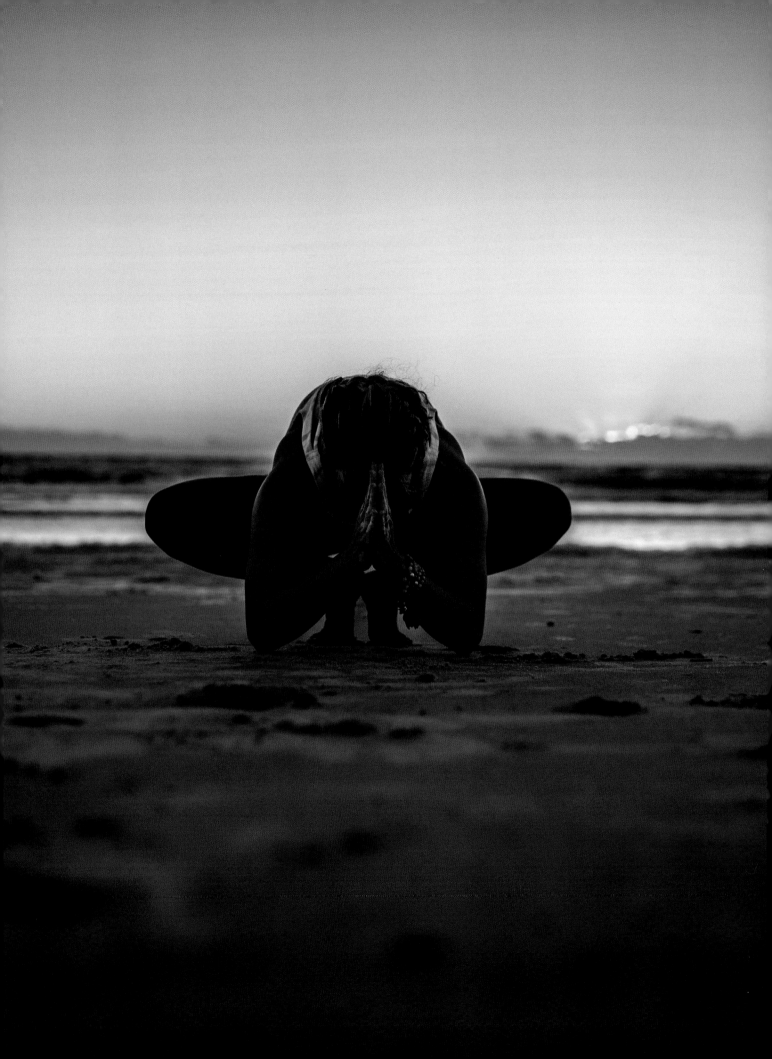

30. THEME: IN SERVICE

When we offer our practice up to something greater than us, we can begin to feel the grandness of what yoga means and the imprint it has, not only on our own lives but also on all the lives we touch, and the ripple effect this causes. I invite you to dedicate this practice to someone or something that resides in your heart or to someone who could use your healing energy.

The other important aspect of offering up our practice outside of ourselves is that it allows us to get out of our own heads a little bit. Maybe in the asana practice we can choose the right modification to show a bit more compassion for someone or something else. Maybe we can discover more strength than we initially thought we possessed, or surrender a bit more than we thought we could. Then the invitation is to carry this intention of service with you off the mat. How can you think, breathe, speak, and act in ways that are in service to someone or something close to your heart?

How does one choose just one dedication? Sometimes I say, "Choose the first person who comes to mind. That's the right one." And then you can allow it to change throughout the practice. Perhaps, "This Warrior II is for my grandfather, who sacrificed everything to emigrate from Hungary to Canada." "This Mountain Pose is for my mom, who taught me to be steady and strong." "This Shiva Dancer is for my dad, for his gift of playfulness and the ability to find balance in the imbalance." "This Vinyasa is for all my students, who always show up with a smile and continue to express gratitude despite all that life throws at them." "This Savasana is for all my teachers and their teachers who have brought this yoga practice to me and so many others; what an amazing blessing!" "I offer this entire practice to my mom for a successful surgery on her spine." "I take with me off the mat a dedication to all the lives affected by this global pandemic."

VIDEO: <u>In Service</u>

PLAYLIST: <u>Be the Change</u>

FEATURED SONG: "<u>Be the Change" by DJ Taz Rashid</u>

HIGHLIGHTED POSE/TRANSITION: Child's Pose with palms facing up.

JOURNAL PROMPT: *How do you offer your yoga practice in service to others?*

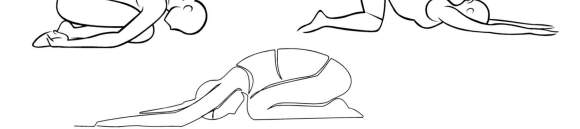

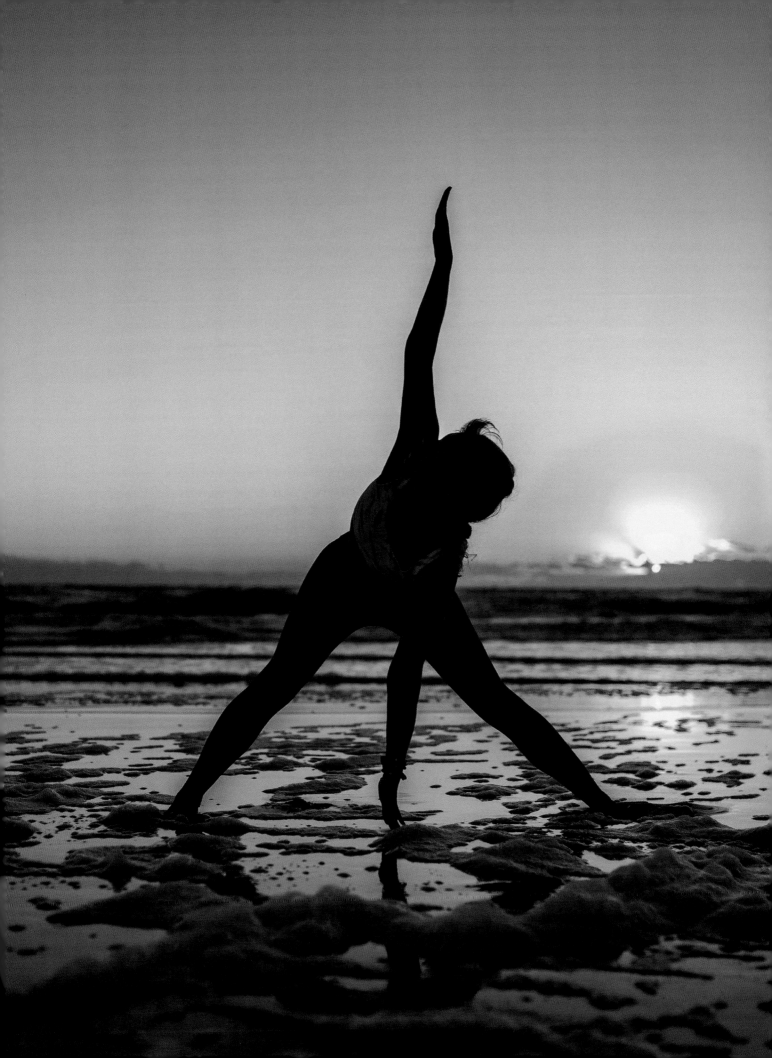

31. THEME: LISTEN IN

Tune in to the body here and now. Tune in to the mind here and now. Listen to your breath. Listen to your heartbeat. Listen to the sounds in your space. Listen to all the information you are receiving through all of your senses.

As we link breath with movement, we can discover what the body is doing in space, what the breath is doing, and what the mind is saying So, we begin this week with movement to shake off the restlessness and open up the channels in the body. Then we come into some long holds to stretch the body and prepare the mind for meditation. Then we come to stillness. The invitation is to close practice in a seated meditation or surrender into your Savasana.

One of my favorite practices these days is turning on music I love and moving my body. Sometimes that looks like dancing around my house and sometimes that looks like free flow on my mat. When I am flowing on my mat, I play with this idea of getting out of my head, getting out of my own way. It's less about creating a sequence per se and more about moving in a way that feels cathartic. I let go of necessarily doing the same thing on each side with more traditional movements, and it truly feels more like my own modern dance.

I used to prefer practicing at night, mostly because I tended to sleep from 2:00 a.m. to 10:00 a.m. in those days. Now I realize if I don't move my body in the morning, I have less energy (and motivation) to do so in the evening. This is another way to tune into yourself. Are you able to take some time to experiment with practicing at different times of day and listening to when your body is happiest? This could also change from day to day if you're sick or feeling emotional. We can choose a habit and then be compassionate with ourselves. The practice is less about movement and more about self-study. What do you need in this moment? Listen in and choose one action to bring you closer.

VIDEO: <u>Listen In</u>

PLAYLIST: <u>Inspiration</u>

FEATURED SONG: <u>"Look inside Yourself" by Edvard Kravchuk</u>

HIGHLIGHTED POSE/TRANSITION: Movement within shapes.

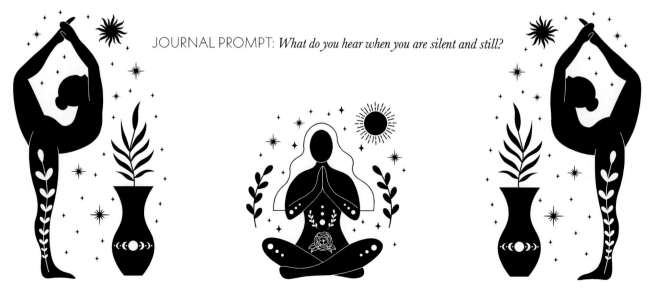

JOURNAL PROMPT: *What do you hear when you are silent and still?*

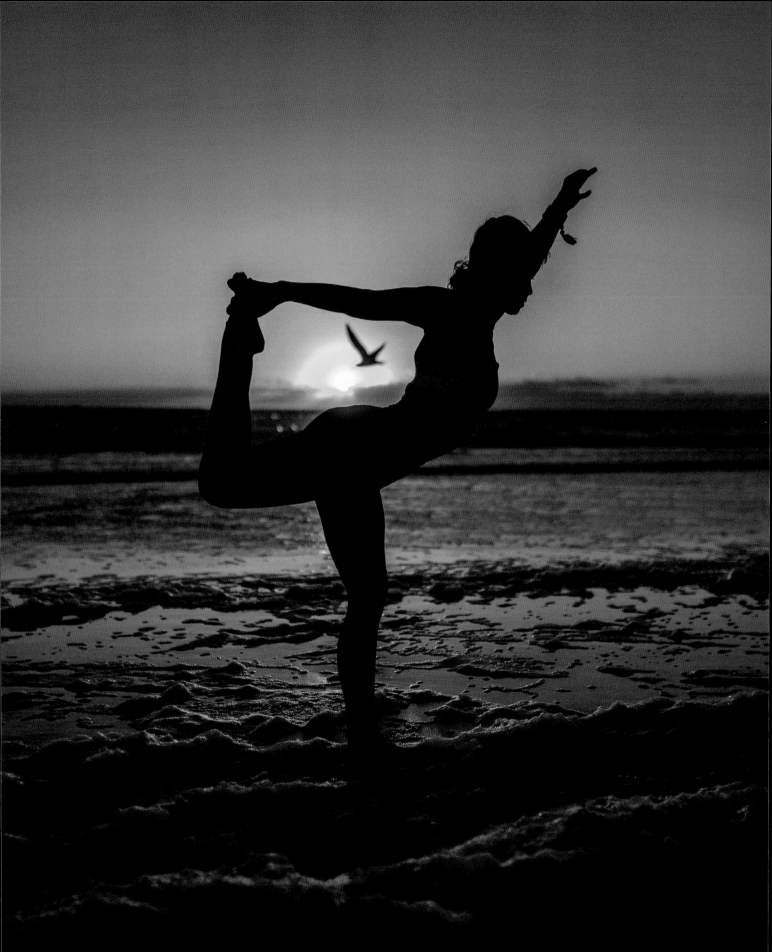

32. THEME: THE MAGIC OF TREES

Whenever I find myself in the woods, I feel a deep connection to the earth and to my breath. In fact, I find I breathe more clearly and peacefully just feeling the energy of the trees nearby. As I write this I am in the Smoky Mountains on a reunion/retreat full of yoga, hiking, rafting, and zip-lining. I love outdoor activities and find that my yoga practice outdoors is integral to finding greater calm and ease in my days. Visualization can be instrumental in guiding our internal world to a meditative state. Close your eyes and feel yourself surrounded by trees. Feel their grounding energy and their assistance in your breath. Embody their poise and their constant growth.

This reunion/retreat has been soul nourishing! I have reunited with the yoga practitioners and instructors from my very first yoga teacher training in Costa Rica through Amazing Yoga, and it has been amazing! Sometimes you meet people for one week in your life in the jungle and you know they are going to be in your life always. That yoga teacher training was one of those times, and these are those people!

We are here in the Smoky Mountains in a cabin on a beautiful hill overlooking the vastness of the fall foliage. Every day has been magic! We take turns leading class for everyone. We all got COVID tests beforehand, so distancing was unnecessary. It felt nice to hug, reunite, and give and receive hands-on assists. I cried in pigeon, like you do when all the emotions are on the surface and your friend comes over and lovingly guides you deeper in the shape. I cried leading the last class of the week while reading out of Melody Beattie's *Journey to the Heart*, just like we did in our yoga teacher training.

One day we decided to wake up at 2:00 a.m. to hike Mt. Cammerer so we could be at the top for sunrise. It seemed like a solid group decision at the time, but the actual act of getting dressed and packed for a hike in the middle of the night had me questioning my sanity. There we were, wearing headlamps in the pitch-black forest, surrounded by bears and snakes, and all we could see was one step in front of us. I'll tell you what: before this hike, I regarded myself as a fit person. During this hike? Not so much. I had to press my hands into my thighs as the incline was so great it felt like I was on a never-ending rugged Stairmaster. Then, somehow, we made it to the top just as the sun was rising, and I had goose bumps. How did I get to be so lucky to be standing on the top of this mountain at sunrise with these beautiful souls?

VIDEO: <u>The Magic of Trees</u>
PLAYLIST: <u>Tree by the River</u>
FEATURED SONG: <u>"Tree by the River" by Iron & Wine</u>

HIGHLIGHTED POSE/TRANSITION: Tree pose!

JOURNAL PROMPT: *Who supports/grounds you?*

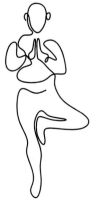

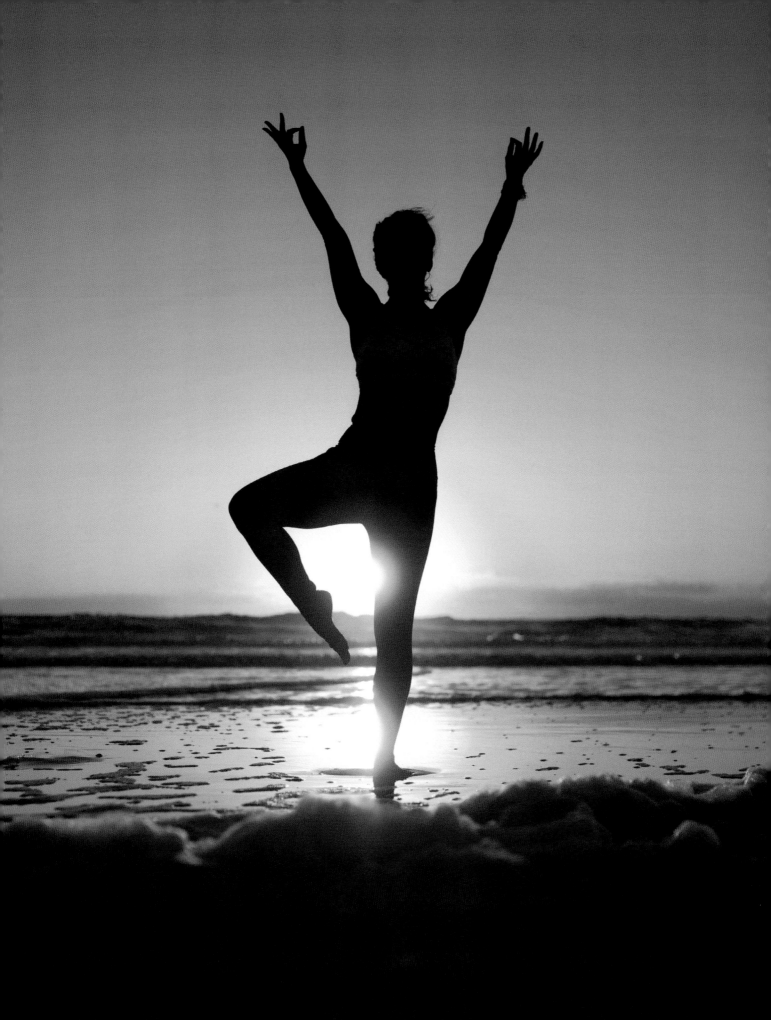

33. THEME: CELEBRATION

Amidst all that's been going on, let's celebrate anyway! Like most people, when I was a kid, I would celebrate my birthday, but these days, I celebrate my birth month. My dad says that when I get older I'll celebrate every day. With that in mind, let's move our bodies, shake things up, and tune back in to all we have to celebrate in our lives.

Think of one, two, three, or many things you can celebrate right now. Breathe those in and breathe them out. Think of one, two, three, or many things you celebrated when you were a child. Are there any similarities between what you celebrated then and what you celebrate now? Think of one, two, three, or many words to align then and now. Let those words become a mantra for you. So, for example, now and then I celebrate fun surprises and that brings me joy. My mantra for this would be "I am joy!" When external circumstances get dark and weighty, I invite you to come back to your mantra. Let it bring you back to this space of celebration and joy.

When I was approaching my thirtieth birthday, something in my brain told me I should go skydiving to celebrate. The thought behind this was that if I can jump out of a plane, then I can do anything! What better year than thirty to prove to myself that nothing of real consequence is an obstacle in pursuit of my dreams? I asked my friend Kevin if he felt as crazy as I did. He did. So there we were, in Perris, California, with my dad in tow, signing our lives away. We watched a video of a lawyer sitting behind the largest mahogany desk I'd ever seen, going through all the reasons why we should be running out the door. And yet we got suited up to jump anyway. The guy I was strapped to was from Switzerland and had jumped about one hundred times. The fact that he was still alive made me feel a bit more confident. It's a strange feeling to find yourself onboard a perfectly operational plane preparing to jump out. My guy told me to kneel at the edge of the plane's open door. I made the mistake of looking down and he lifted my chin up: "Don't do that."

Next thing I knew, he practically pushed us out of the plane! Suddenly, we were free-falling at a pace of, I don't know, let's say a million miles per hour. He said, "Do you want to pull the parachute chord?"

"Do I want to pull the parachute chord? No, thank you." The expert should be in charge of that! And in less than a second, things went from terrifying to pleasant. Or at least I no longer felt like I was plunging to my death.

My heart was still in my throat when my feet touched the ground. My dad said, "Can we go celebrate now?"

I have the whole ordeal on video because I realized it would be a once-in-a-lifetime affair. I am glad I did it, and it was certainly was one of my most memorable birthdays. That's for sure!

VIDEO: <u>Celebration</u>

PLAYLIST: <u>Baby from 1980</u>

FEATURED SONG: <u>"(Just Like) Starting Over" by John Lennon</u>

HIGHLIGHTED POSE/TRANSITION: Dance party—rock it out and find the moves that move you.

JOURNAL PROMPT: *Describe your most memorable celebratory event or moment.*

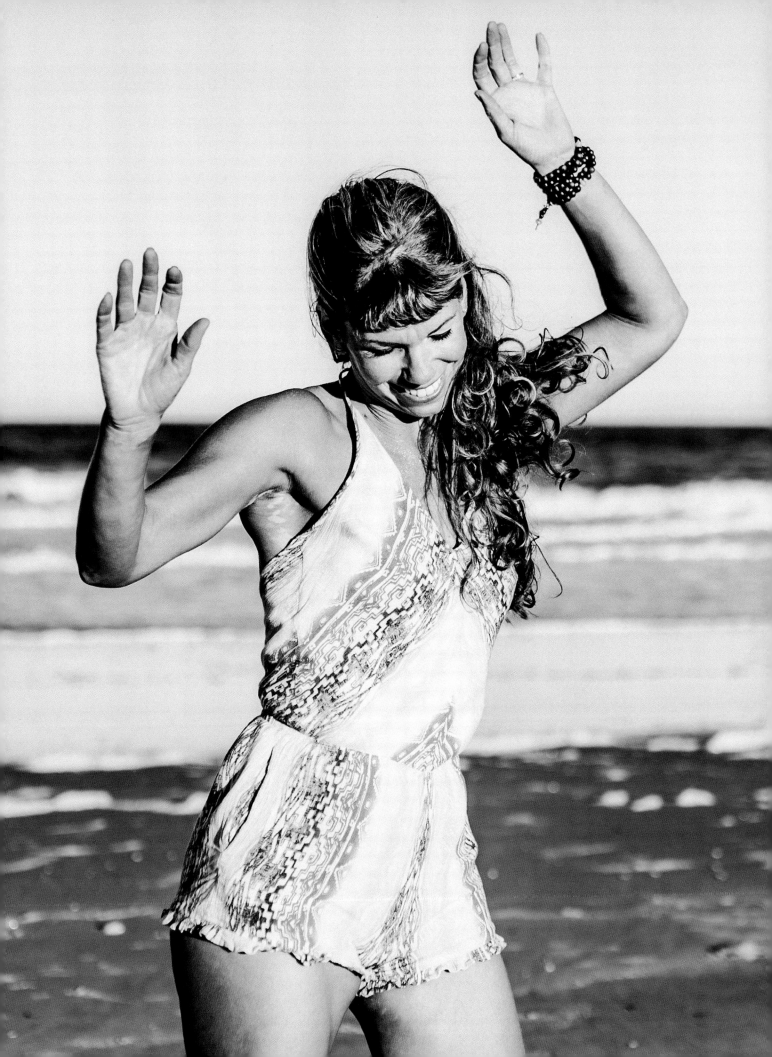

34. THEME: SHARE YOUR VOICE

Open your heart and share your voice in a space that is kind and true. As we unite our breath, we recognize and feel deeply that what unites us is greater than what divides us.

I wrote this theme during election week. My original intention was to encourage everyone to vote. But as the week progressed, and we found ourselves waiting for a final, definitive result, I began to see it as an opportunity for us to notice and observe our triggers. Find four rounds of breath (at least) before responding to someone or something that sets you off, redirecting any knee-jerk reactions. We are living in tumultuous times, but we can choose how much media we consume, which conversations we get wrapped up in, and the tone we observe even in our thoughts. I choose not to share my political views in this setting as my attention is on what connects us rather than what divides us.

We have the opportunity in Camel Pose to open up the throat chakra, representing opening the blockages that prevent us from speaking our truth. Feel inspired to share your voice in truth and kindness.

For Christmas last year, Brandon surprised me with a harmonium, a handcrafted organ instrument from India. I had been enchanted by it since my practices at Pure Yoga West when Dana Slamp and Miles Borrero would chant and invite us to join in. I had the idea to envelop my students with sound in lieu of hands-on assists, providing a soundscape, particularly for my Yin Deep Stretch classes while my students were holding a shape.

With the advent of Zoom, I was able to take harmonium lessons with both Dana and Miles. I told them individually of my plans to simply play. While I love to sing and chant, I don't have a professional singer's voice. But they both independently heard me and invited me to learn a chant anyway. With their encouragement, I thought perhaps I might lead my students to Om.

Two weeks into my lessons, Dana said, "Your homework is to bring the harmonium to class and guide your students out of Savasana with a couple of simple chords and then guide them to Om." I was nervous and hesitant! Dana and Miles have amazing singing voices and it all felt a bit intimidating. Plus, as far as I knew, no one in Vero Beach played the harmonium or guided chants in yoga classes. I wasn't sure how it would be received. As soon as I walked into the studio with my harmonium in tow that Saturday, one of my students saw it right away, and with excitement asked, "Are we going to chant?" I heard myself saying, "Yes!" I guided my students through Dana Slamp's Lokah Samastah Sukino Bhavantu chant. I sang, my students sang, and it was a beautiful union of voices. It felt palpable, the power of sharing your voice and inviting my students to share their voices, all of us sharing the message:

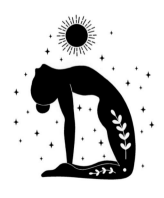

may my actions contribute to the happiness of all
may my actions contribute to the freedom of all
not me alone, not me alone
Om

VIDEO: <u>Share Your Voice</u>
PLAYLIST: <u>Awake Me</u>
FEATURED SONG: <u>"Follow My Voice"</u> by <u>Julie Byrne</u>

HIGHLIGHTED POSE/TRANSITION: Camel Pose.

JOURNAL PROMPT: *Write down all the things you want to say.*

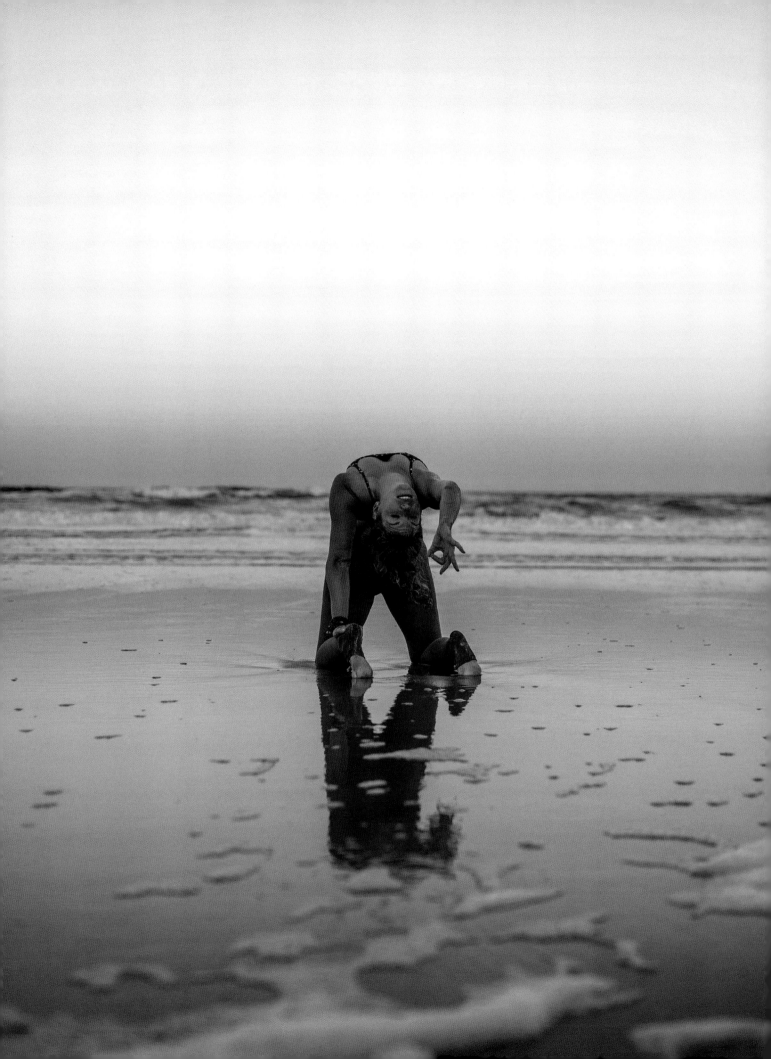

35. THEME: ROOT CHAKRA

Breathe in a feeling of home, safe and sound. When do you feel most grounded, secure, tethered, and anchored? As we draw our awareness to the base of the spine and the pelvic floor and focus our attention on our connection to the earth, we can begin to harness our own ability to find balance at our root chakra. And when we focus on one part of the body, it becomes another meditation tool for the mind to focus on, tethering us to the here and now.

Meditate on when you feel most grounded. Who are you with? Are you alone? Where are you? What are you wearing? What are the smells in your space? Are you cozy and tranquil or out and active? Visualize yourself in your perfect scene of feeling grounded. Paint all the colors and experience it as it is happening in this moment. Breathe with this for ten breaths, slow and steady. Now, what word or words would you use to encapsulate your visualization? I invite you to use this word or words as a mantra throughout your week, letting this rooting feeling live in you regardless of where you are, who you are with, or what situation you are in. Discover your inner world of feeling grounded.

My feeling of what grounding means to me has shifted over the years. I used to feel more anchored when I was surrounded by friends (read: only child syndrome). I remember when I was fourteen years old, I'd love to host all my friends at my house every day possible! My lawn would be covered in bikes and we would hang out in the basement, playing Nintendo and ping-pong, and plotting out how to sneak out and into the neighborhood pool after hours.

These days, oh my, how I do relish my time alone! I yearn for it and I need it to feel charged. I love the silence, the tranquility of simple practices by myself.

Do you know *The Home Edit* series on Netflix? It's great! It's all about putting things into containers. You might be wondering how this relates to the grounding practice. I find tremendous peace and feel most at balance when my home is organized and tidy. So on a study break last week, I emptied all the contents of my pantry. This was an epic project! I essentially did my own "home edit." All the food is now beautifully organized in containers with labels on them and you can see everything at a glance. If you want a quick preview of the kind of organization I'm talking about, I suggest stalking The Home Edit's Instagram page. Sometimes I'll open the pantry door and just look at how lovely everything looks now and I truly feel more anchored and peaceful.

VIDEO: <u>Root Chakra</u>

PLAYLIST: <u>Grounded</u>

FEATURED SONG: <u>"Root Chakra" by Beautiful Chorus</u>

HIGHLIGHTED POSE/TRANSITION: Malasana.

JOURNAL PROMPT: *Describe when you feel most grounded.*

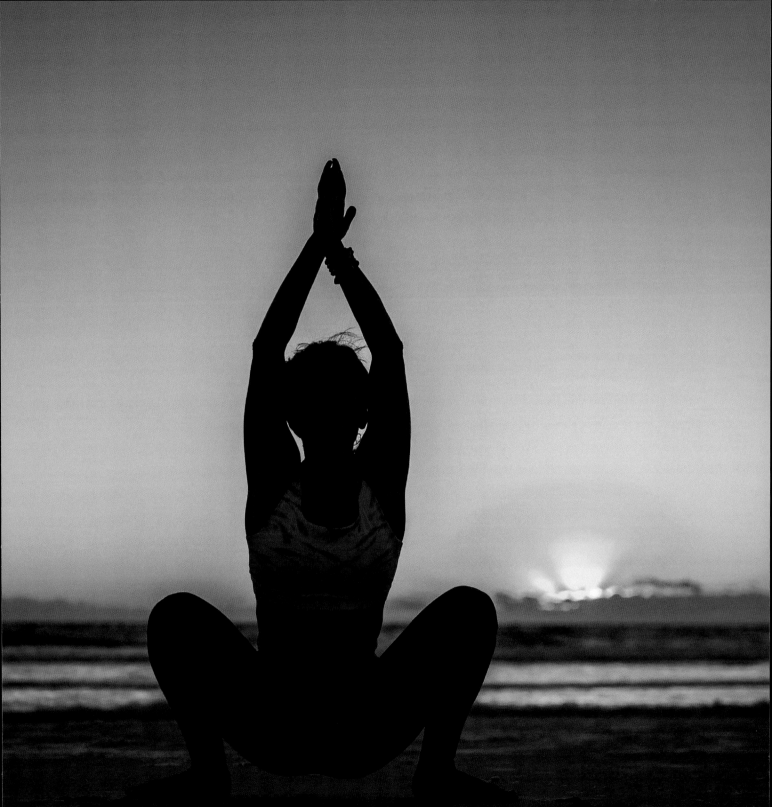

36. THEME: SACRAL CHAKRA

How did you express your creativity when you were ten years old? How do you express your creativity now? Do elements of your childhood expressions remain today? As we explore our sacral chakra, our space of creativity, we come into alignment with feeling vibrant. We can ignite this light within through visualization. Our imagination can spark our inner artist. We can also inspire our creative impulses by moving the body in new ways. Come into an expression of yourself that feels true.

Imagine a beautiful orange light within you. Let it fill you up with each inhale and let it wash away with each exhale. Imagine your inner world painted like a watercolor with the use of your breath. Let this inner artist thrive with attention to inner focus.

Take this springboard of expression with you throughout your day and week. Let your light shine through writing, visual art, performance art, dance, music, cooking, gardening, or creating something new.

Both of my grandmothers were artists. My mom's mom was a gifted painter. I have some of her paintings in my house and feel her presence there. My dad's mom was a phenomenal cook and baker, and she was also skilled in fabrics, specializing in custom drapes and curtains. Being exposed to these talents as a young child inspired me. I don't have the natural patience for cooking or painting, but I do enjoy these artistic expressions when I set out to do them.

About ten years ago, my mom, aunt, uncle, and I went on an Alaskan cruise. We were the punch line of the stand-up comic on board. "Only Canadians would choose to cruise in Alaska in the summer!" The glaciers were incredible! (So was the hot cocoa with Bailey's.) One of the activities on board (and you know I love activities) was a painting class. The teachers guided us to create beautiful snowcapped mountain peaks in watercolor. They taught us to keep the empty spaces, allowing them to become the snow. The mountains themselves could be multicolored or any color we chose. I painted mine in blues and purples. I enjoyed creating those mountains with the snowy peaks. I still have this painting. I keep it on my fridge. It reminds me, not just of that vacation, but also that creating something is fuel for the self.

VIDEO: <u>Sacral Chakra</u>

PLAYLIST: <u>Inspiration</u>

FEATURED SONG: <u>"Inspiration" by Freedom Fry</u>

HIGHLIGHTED POSES/TRANSITIONS: Creative movement
within a shape and unique explorations in transitions.

JOURNAL PROMPT: *What and who inspires you?*

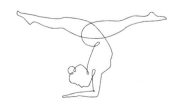

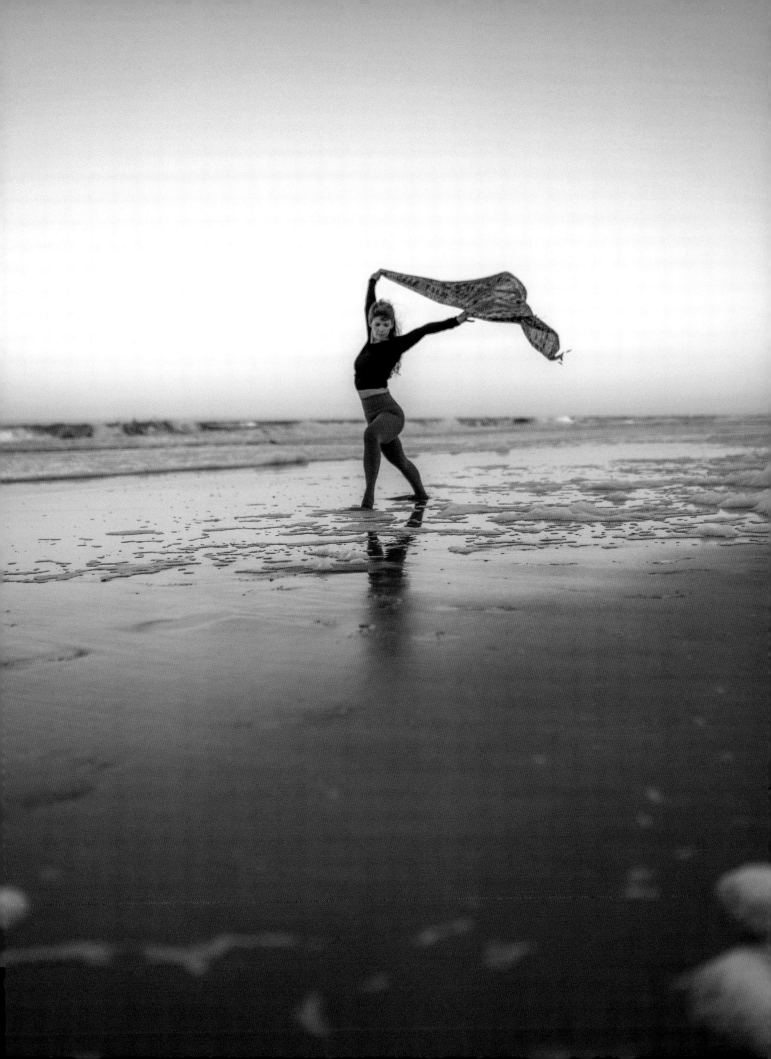

37. THEME: SOLAR PLEXUS CHAKRA

It likely is no coincidence that we arrive at the solar plexus chakra during the week of Thanksgiving. Our entry point above the naval will be accessed through twists stimulating our digestion. When we are in balance here, we are in our power and exhibiting warrior energy. How better to access our strength than to wring out physical toxins and toxic thoughts so we can arrive with unabashed confidence?

Breathe in the color yellow to the space above the naval. Feel the sun fill you up and light a fire from within. When do you feel powerful? Who do you feel powerful with? In what situations do you thrive? How can you embody and exude this energy in the here and now? Little by little, you will learn to rely less on external circumstances to dictate a sense of balance within.

First off, please do not feel guilty that you have indulged and eaten so much. A mindfulness practice exists even in overindulgence. If you're going to eat all the turkey, stuffing, green bean casserole, mac and cheese, and the sweet potatoes with the marshmallows, and then get another plate before all the pumpkin pie, enjoy! Honestly and truly! When we make the decision to eat something (or do something), it is far more healing to enjoy it unabashedly than it is to tie our stomachs in knots with thoughts like "I shouldn't be doing this." I know this all too well. Many external influences dictate to us what is "good" or "bad," and one of the lessons I'm letting sink in this year from my Authentic Movements training is: "It depends." Maybe gathering with family and eating a rich meal is just what you need in the moment. Perhaps the next day you feel a bit heavier. Or maybe not. You can decide meal by meal and moment by moment what serves you and what doesn't. Then you can decide, with compassion, to wring out the parts that don't serve. I've discovered that it's usually not the second slice of pumpkin pie, but rather my thoughts or the story I tell myself about having the second slice.

So here we are. We've made the decisions we've made; we've eaten all we've eaten. Warrior I: stand and embrace yourself for all you are. Warrior II: pull the arrow for all the parts of yourself you are letting go. Warrior III: be the arrow and fly free.

Feel and believe your warrior energy is powerfully you!

VIDEO: Solar Plexus Chakra

PLAYLIST: Gratitude

FEATURED SONG: "I Believe in You" by Michael Bublé

HIGHLIGHTED POSES/TRANSITIONS: Twists.

JOURNAL PROMPT: *When and with whom do you feel warrior energy?*

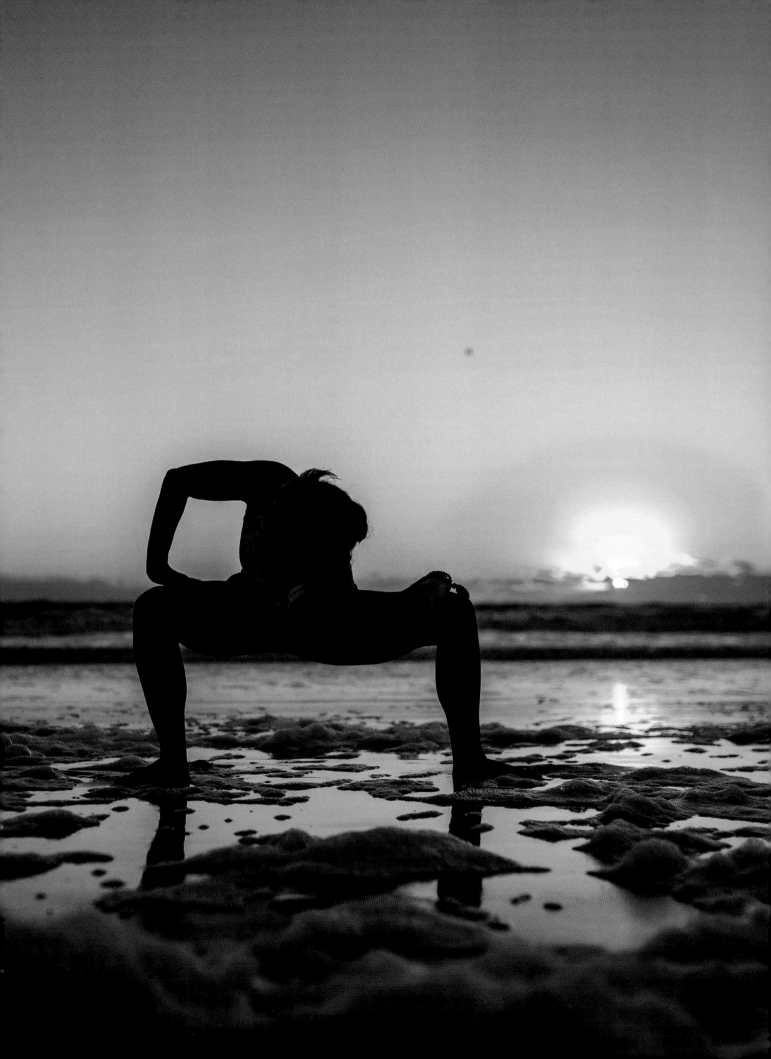

38. THEME: HEART CHAKRA

truly love this week's flow! We found the bow bind on our bellies, in side plank, building dancer's pose from the ground up and finding half-moon with the bind and then flowing from half-moon to Shiva squat with a twist back and forth. We have a lot of opportunities to crack our heart open in this week's flow. With the attention of the breath to the heart, we carve more and more space here with the intention to open ourselves to receive love from ourselves and from others and to give love to all beings.

I realize that the flexibility of each person, as well as one's personal history with back injuries, may make these backbends an opportunity to create more mindfulness surrounding the depth you guide yourself into with these shapes. Additionally, the opening of the heart literally and figuratively is a vulnerable act. So breathe into this moment to discover with truthfulness where you can soften and surrender. Perhaps this is the week to reestablish a "comfortable uncomfortable" and love this moment, this you, and this life, just as it is.

As I mentioned earlier, I love heart openers! And just like all of us, when I love something, I lean in to it. It is just like in our childhood studies, where some of us happened to be good at math and science while others were all about art and language. You can also probably guess which camp I was part of, right? But we can each access an entry point into each shape or subject even if it isn't our forte. For me, though my passion is storytelling and creativity, I've found access into the left brain through learning about anatomy and physiology, as it supports the movement as it applies to my body as well as my students'.

If you're resistant to these heart-opener shapes, this may be an opportunity to tune inward. It may be a physical or emotional inhibition, or maybe it's a learned response. Then, there's this other component that the shape should look a certain way. We can find a heart opener seated and think cow pose in the spine. We could be lying down with a small throw pillow between the shoulder blades. We could be standing with our hands against the wall and allowing the torso to dip below the arms like a supported puppy pose. Or we could think about guiding the breath into the heart space front and back. When you practice what you love, how do you feel? When you practice what you resist, how do you feel? Finding your way to practice into your heart space just might help you crack yourself open to live a life of liberation.

VIDEO: <u>Heart Chakra</u>

PLAYLIST: <u>And I Love Her</u>

FEATURED SONG: <u>"Golden (Acoustic)" by Becca Mancari</u>

HIGHLIGHTED POSES/TRANSITIONS: Attention to the front, back, and sides of the heart. Half-moon pose with the option for a bind.

JOURNAL PROMPT: *What is your heart's intention—for this moment, for this practice, for this life?*

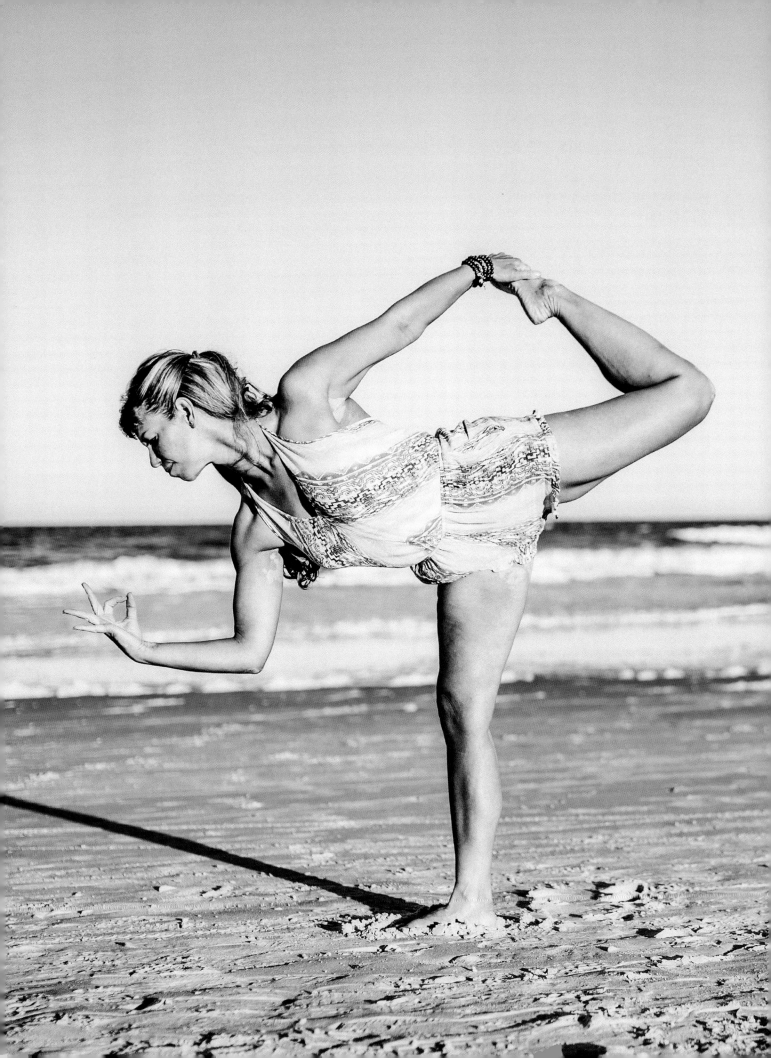

39. THEME: THROAT CHAKRA

Enjoy the symbolism of opening the throat space physically to create space to share your voice. We begin by observing our thoughts and asking ourselves, "Is it true? Is it kind? Is it necessary?" When our throat chakra is in balance, we speak our truth in the space of loving-kindness. When our throat chakra is out of balance, we may gossip, be silent, or speak harshly.

So let's explore a way to open not only the front of the throat but also the sides and back of the neck. We'll also extend to open up the shoulders, the hips, and the feet. Notice where there is resistance in the body and where there is flow. Try to observe the openness and the tension without judgment. Breathe loving-kindness to the body and breathe loving-kindness to the thoughts. When the physical body is challenged, notice when the mind tells you that you can't do something. Remark on how you create that reality with your thoughts. Trust the strength of your mind and your body. You are stronger than you know.

Over the years, I've had students share with me their feelings of depression. Through the yoga and meditation practices, I've had these same students share how they have started to change their thought patterns from self-hatred to self-love. There is a lot of science, research, and studies to support this powerful mind and reality shift.

It makes sense that we should concentrate not merely on avoiding negative emotions, like fear and anger, but also on consciously cultivating heartfelt, positive emotions, such as gratitude, joy, excitement, enthusiasm, fascination, awe, inspiration, wonder, trust, appreciation, kindness, compassion, and empowerment to give us every advantage in maximizing our health. —Dr. Joe Dispenza, *Evolve Your Brain: The Science of Changing Your Mind*

One way to begin shifting our thoughts is through the practice of observation. When we become attuned to the thoughts that arrive, we can begin assessing if they are true, or if we perceive them as true. Oftentimes it is challenging to delineate our perceived truth from concrete truth. Asking the question of ourselves is paramount in shifting the way we talk to ourselves. Try to observe without judgment and practice the opposite and see how you feel. For example, if the thought is "I hate myself," try on "I love myself." Repeat and repeat again.

VIDEO: <u>Throat Chakra</u>

PLAYLIST: <u>Say Something</u>

FEATURED SONG: <u>"Say Something" by Guitar Tribute Players</u>

HIGHLIGHTED POSE/TRANSITION: Fish pose.

JOURNAL PROMPT: *What is something you need to say for yourself or to someone else?*

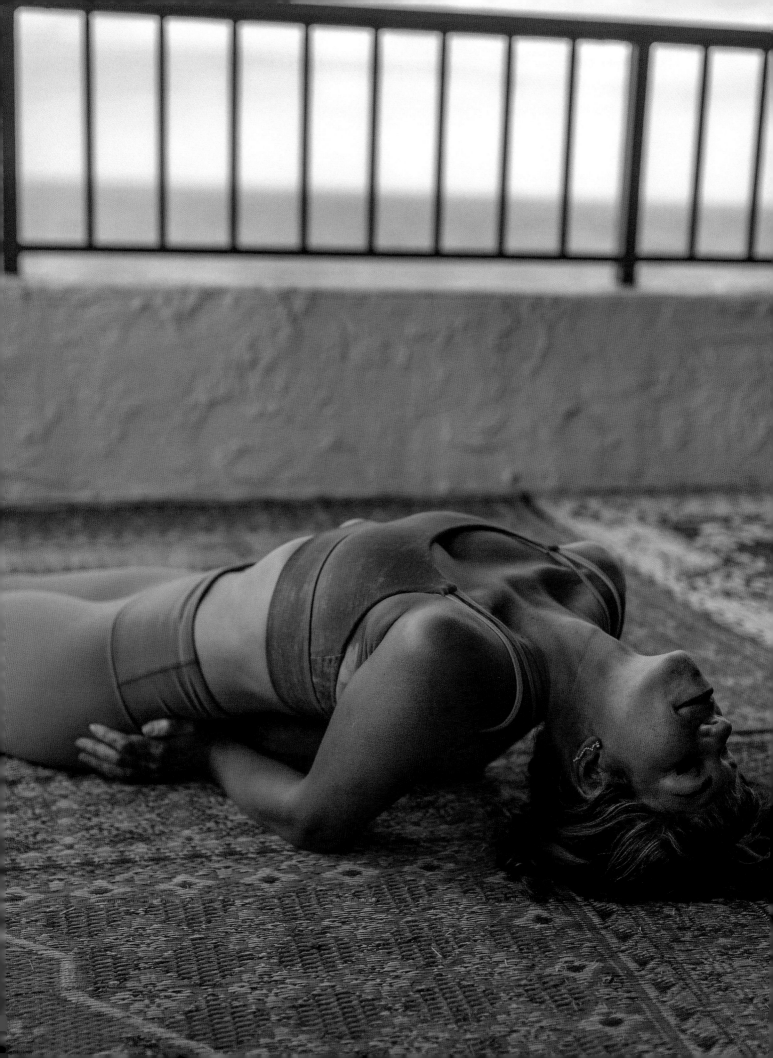

40. THEME: THIRD EYE CHAKRA

Begin in child's pose, resting your third eye to the earth or onto a block. Find a physical connection to your third eye space as a portal to connect to your own inner gaze, your intuition. Bow your head to the earth as a gesture to invite the mind to step to the side, allowing your heart and your gut to guide you. Visualize a gorgeous indigo light at the third eye, calming you and encouraging you to trust in yourself. This flow is sequenced to stimulate your third eye, your space of intuition. It is transformative to witness how our awareness of our own thoughts can cultivate tremendous shifts in the way we allow ourselves to be guided.

Sometimes that intuitive ping in the gut, heart, brain, or wherever it hits you taps, taps, taps. I have been known to ignore it because logic, circumstance, or something else needs to take its course. In hindsight, I would say I ignored my intuition for seventeen years. This isn't to say that I regret those years and all I learned and all I was able to create; however, I do wonder where I would be if I had trusted myself more at twenty-two years old.

During the very first Athena Theatre production, it felt like everything went wrong. This chronicle could likely be its own book. We scheduled auditions through agents and managers at a location where I took classes. When we arrived, the owner acted as though he couldn't remember our conversation and said we couldn't hold auditions there. Because we were in LA, where everything is spread out, we pivoted quickly to the Barnes & Noble café. We thought, "At least we can meet with everyone and have an initial conversation." Then the manager came over. "Are you holding auditions in my café?" (Perhaps I should have mentioned that, in the rush, we didn't actually ask permission. Oops.)

We found ourselves standing on the wheelchair ramp outside of the Barnes & Noble café pretending to be professionals. Fast-forward a few weeks to rehearsals. My costar, who was a dream the whole rehearsal process (Did I mention this was a two person show?), decided that, because the character is drunk in the scene, he too must be drunk. So he put real gin in the prop bottle, which I also drank from, then proceeded to ignore all the blocking (staged movement), and threw a (prop) knife at me, causing me to stumble backward into one of the walls, which then fell on me. Luckily, we had had the foresight to cast understudies! The understudy went on and did the whole run and somehow I forgot all the craziness and we produced show after show after show.

There were red flags like this throughout the seventeen years, but I think my heart kept telling my brain to shut the fuck up. As an eternal optimist, I thought it would get better once we got more money or had more history behind us. And eventually, that tap, tap, tap of intuition became a sledgehammer. I knew it was time to make what would be one of the hardest decisions of my life. When I moved to Florida, I continued to run my company remotely and our last year was our fullest season in our history! I flew to NYC for our last production. It was the NYC premiere of *I Carry Your Heart* by Georgette Kelly at the Off-Broadway venue 59E59 Theaters. A designer had left the show a week before we opened, and producing the show with the original vision seemed utterly impossible. I stood on the sidewalk with my dear friend and associate producer, Chris, trying to figure out what we were doing. It was very emotional for me. I poured everything I had into this company and the struggle to thrive felt insurmountable. I said to Chris, "I can't continue like this." I began to cry. We refer to this conversation as the moment of clarity, standing on the sidewalk on the Upper East Side with a mountain of trash bags piled up next to us and the sounds of the city buzzing all around us. This was the beginning of the decision, but I didn't know it yet.

VIDEO: <u>Third Eye Chakra</u>
PLAYLIST: <u>Inspiration</u>
FEATURED SONG: <u>"Look Inside Yourself"</u> by Edvard Kravchuk

HIGHLIGHTED POSE/TRANSITION: Warrior III with head resting on forearm, opposite arm alongside the body.

JOURNAL PROMPT: *Do you follow your intuition?*

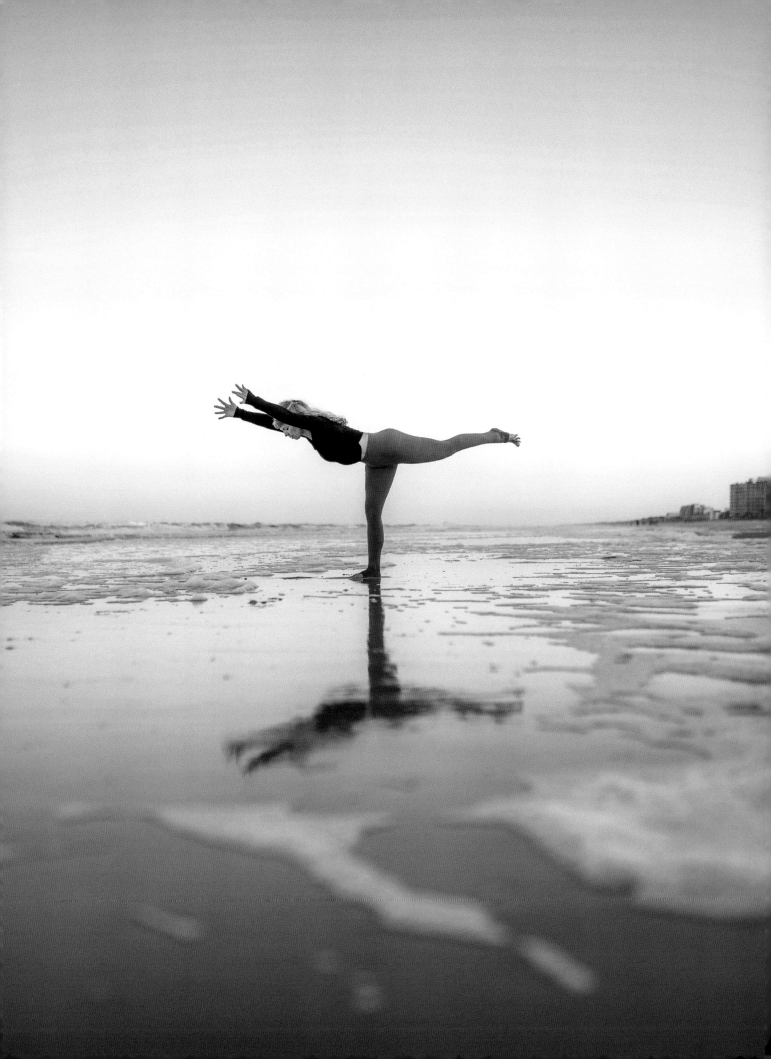

41. THEME: CROWN CHAKRA

How do we feel a sense of fulfillment in the here and now, just as we are? There is an opportunity to practice contentment with what is. How do we do this? As we focus on the crown chakra space, the space of spirituality and fulfillment, perhaps we could entertain the notion that everything is as it should be. As we continue to learn and strive, to be the best version of ourselves on this day and in the here and now—even though we embrace that there is much yet to learn and spaces to grow into—there is solace in knowing that this version of ourselves in the here and now is enough as well. This practice of achieving fulfillment can be felt in each asana shape—from left side to right side—from today to twenty years ago. This is a practice of nonattachment, certainly to how the shape looks and also to how it feels.

I recently hosted a three-day headstand challenge. Headstand isn't for everyone certainly, and other shapes, accessible for all bodies, stimulate the crown chakra. But often fear gets in the way. I know it did for me and I had some false starts to my yoga practice. It wasn't until 2012, when I found the right studio and the right teachers for me, that I began practicing daily (shout-out to The Yoga Room in Astoria, Queens!). I began humbly, curious, a bit intimidated, but overall inspired.

There was a yoga contest in the first year or two of my practice where you had to submit a photo of yourself in a yoga pose. I had recently found headstand against the wall, and I was super proud of myself. Granted, I was not very solid at the wall, but I could find the shape. The photo turned out blurry because I was moving a little, but I love that photo. To me, it represents courage.

I never thought I'd be brave enough to break up with "Paul the Wall" (Paul the Wall is like an on-again, off-again boyfriend: He's helpful sometimes, but at other times he's just a crutch). But with the help of teachers spotting me and practicing a lot, I finally got there.

These more complex shapes take time. Enjoy the little wins along the way. I know sometimes it's easy to focus on the big wins, but it takes a very many little wins to get there. Please be sweet and patient with yourself.

VIDEO: <u>Crown Chakra</u>

PLAYLIST: <u>Opening</u>

FEATURED SONG: <u>"The Call" by Regina Spektor</u>

HIGHLIGHTED POSES/TRANSITIONS: **Hare or Headstand.**

JOURNAL PROMPT: *Write down all you need to feel fulfilled. Circle one and journal the feeling this represents. How can you achieve this sense of fulfillment this week?*

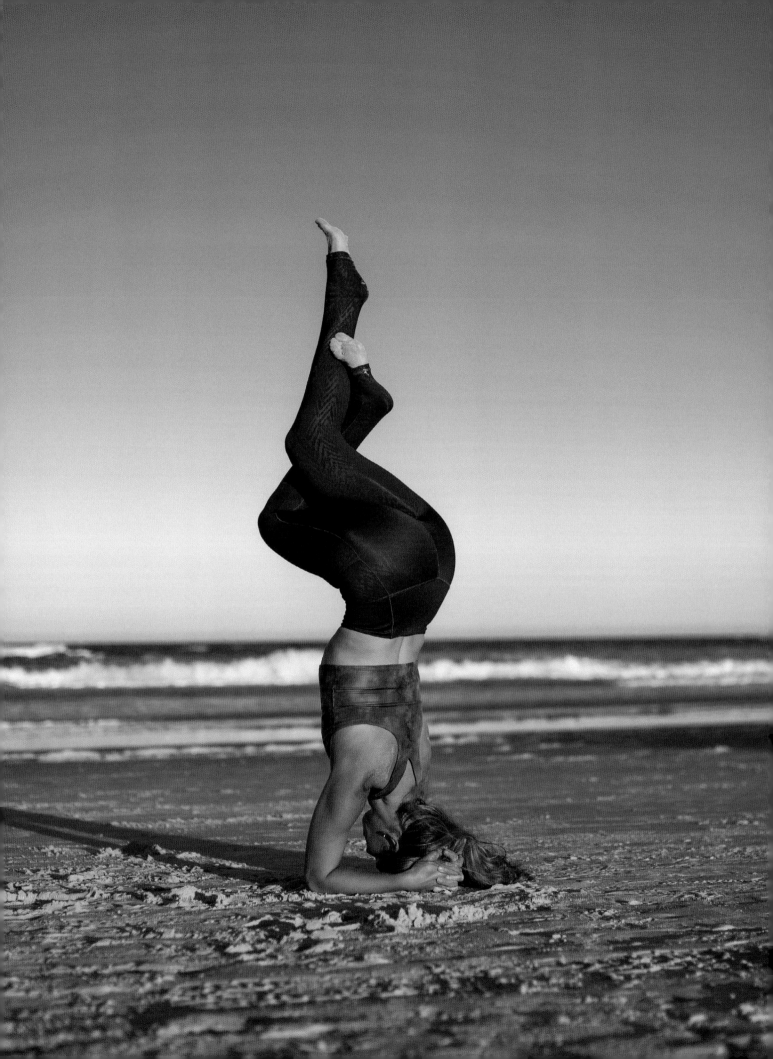

42. THEME: BEGINNER'S MIND

t's the beginning of a new year! Happy New Year!!! And what better time to explore beginner's mind than when we arrive at a new year? Before we come into this new year, I invite you to move your body, shake your body out, and release any residual attachments to yesteryear. Then come into Mountain Pose. Place one hand to your belly and one hand to your heart and feel your breath, your heart, and your energetic pulsations.

In the beginner's mind there are many possibilities, but in the expert's there are few. —Shunryu Suzuki, *Zen Mind, Beginner's Mind*

Step into this moment with this in mind. What if you did not know what was to come, what your body is capable of, or how your mind typically patterns through thoughts? Here we can take the Etch A Sketch of our previous habits, shake it up to clear the slate, and arrive with the mindset of wonderment.

Choose a New Year's resolution and shift the phrasing in your mind to be an affirmation. For example, if your New Year's resolution is "I'm going to be calm this year," change it to "I am calm." Look at your resolution too to see if, instead of telling yourself what you won't do or shouldn't do, you can shift that to an action you want to do. For example, shift "I'm not going to be anxious" to "I am calm."

If you'd like a phenomenal guided New Year's intention-setting ritual, I highly recommend visiting *The Yoga Girl* podcast, "Conversations from the Heart" by Rachel Brathen: "The light you are seeking is within your own heart."

VIDEO: <u>Beginner's Mind</u>

PLAYLIST: <u>Hope</u>

FEATURED SONG: <u>"Rays of Hope" by Oneke</u>

HIGHLIGHTED POSES/TRANSITIONS: Explorations of shapes from a different perspective or using props to discover a different access to a shape.

JOURNAL PROMPT: *Write down your New Year's affirmation. Write down the one you are called to, not the one you think you should have. Once you have your heart's affirmation, write it down boldly and place this affirmation where you can see it every day.*

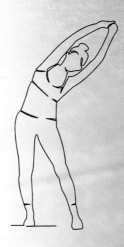

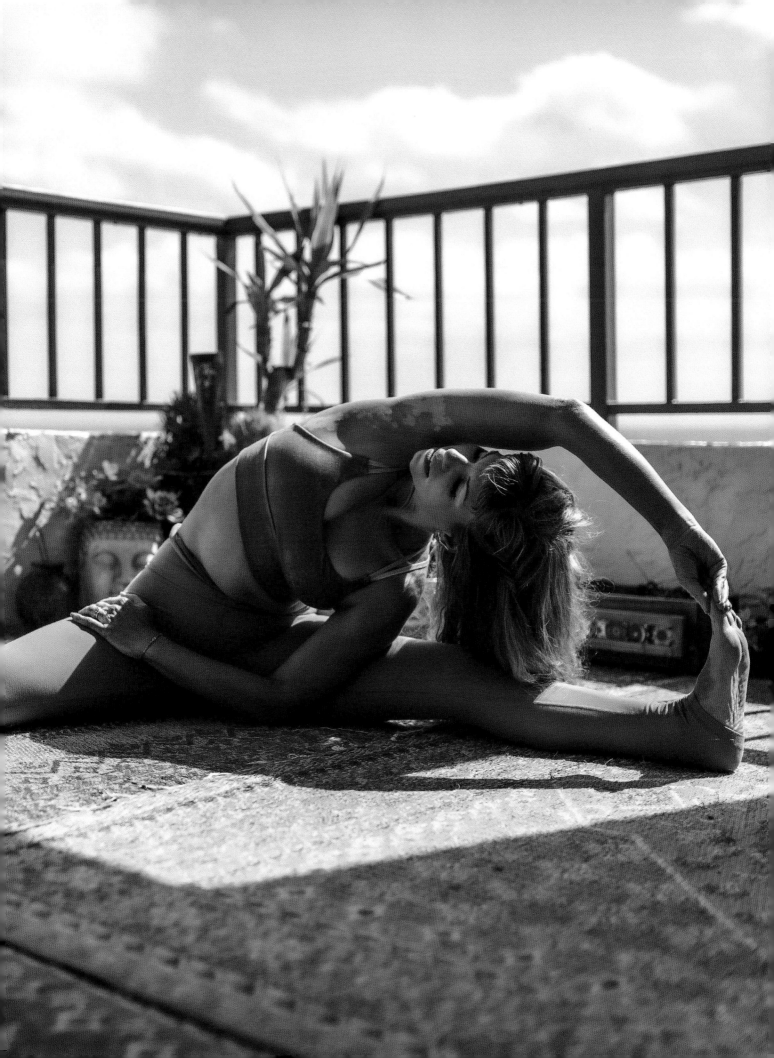

43. THEME: BE A YES

"Be a Yes" is the first philosophy from Baptiste Yoga. We can interpret this philosophy in different ways. Oftentimes, we may assume that "being a yes" means saying yes all of the time. Sometimes "being a yes" means saying no. We may sometimes get caught up in agreeing to more than we want to or are capable of, for fear of letting others down or because we assume we have more energy than we actually do.

I like this theme as a sort of scaffolding for this week's practice to examine your awareness of when your mind, body, and soul are in complete agreement of a YES! We get to practice this shape to shape, breath to breath, variation to variation. This is a portal into the self off the mat. We come back to this concept of filling our own cup first so we can be of service to others. Awaken your awareness to when your yes is serving your higher self, your ego, others, your assumptions of what must be done, or simply old habits. Wipe the slate clean and breathe into your yes of the now!

A very silly memory comes to mind from when I lived with my friend Matt in NYC. Whenever I would find myself debating something, whether it was to pursue a project or buy a dress, he would say, "If it's not a hell yes, it's a hell no." It makes me smile when I hear his voice saying this. It helps with my decision-making process. Sometimes, of course, it's more complicated. In those situations, my dad would lovingly spend hours on the phone with me creating pros and cons lists. Then we would attach a value to each item on the list, because maybe there's only one item on the pro list and ten on the con list, but the one item on the pro list is worth a lot more. (Of course, only the one with the task of making the decision can determine the value.) Then my dad would tell me to throw away the list and act as if I'd made the decision. "How do you feel?" he would ask. It's amazing how illuminating this role play often was! Oftentimes, even though the internal debate can be heated, the simple act of deciding and sitting back and seeing how it lands is so liberating. Now, what if each time you are considering yes or no, you are acting in a way to live your most vibrant life, whatever that means to you?

VIDEO: <u>Be a Yes</u>

PLAYLIST: <u>Be the Change</u>

FEATURED SONG: <u>"Heart Sutra" by Wah!</u>

HIGHLIGHTED POSE/TRANSITION: Happy baby.

JOURNAL PROMPT: *What does "being a yes" mean to you? What must be in alignment in your life to feel like your yes is fully expressed?*

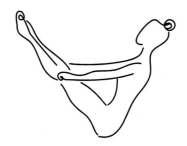

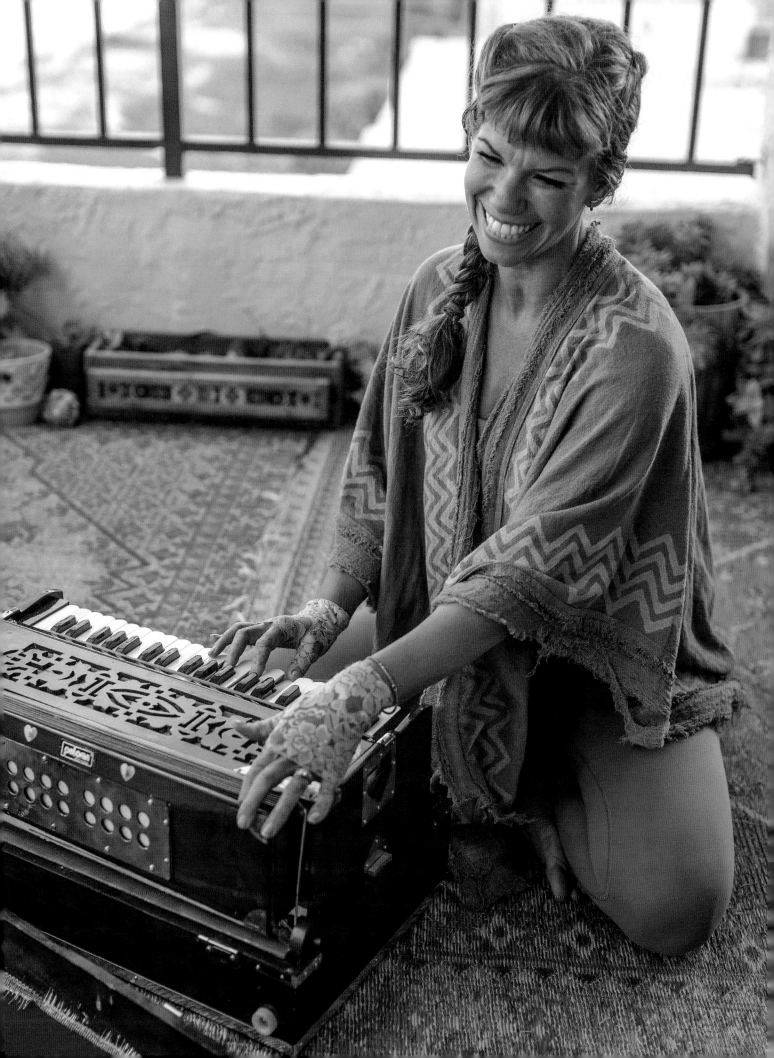

44. THEME: GIVE UP WHAT YOU MUST

When we think of purging or letting go, we may initially think in the realm of physical stuff or material possessions. But we can also think in terms of self-image, self-limiting beliefs, what we assume our body is or isn't capable of, what we think we can achieve, old physical or emotional wounds, or the roles we've assigned ourselves or have had assigned to us, whether in our family or among our close friends. Even though something is a habit and perhaps can even feel "fine," it is worth examining whether these habits, these thoughts, or, yes, these physical objects, are elevating you to your highest purpose.

We can visualize our lives, our houses, our spaces, and our every day. Zoom out and look objectively at all that you need and all that might be superfluous. Awaken to a new day with a fresh perspective: change is not only possible, it allows for countless other possibilities. When we carve out the space from the things that no longer serve, we invite space in our lives for the things that do serve. So break up with your ego and your self-doubt for a moment and see before you your life realized with beauty, peace, love, kindness, abundance, joy, and fulfillment.

When I let go of what I am, I become what I might be. When I let go of what I have, I receive what I need. —Lao Tzu

The practice of nonattachment is a very challenging one for me. I form attachments to people, places, things, a certain way of being, my schedule, or the expectations I've set for myself or for any given situation, very easily. Yet I see so much change in practically every facet of life and I have only just recently become friendly with the practice of letting go. It's vulnerable and scary and uncomfortable. But I also feel a tremendous freedom and liberation on the other side.

VIDEO: <u>Give Up What You Must</u>

PLAYLIST: <u>Reflection</u>

FEATURED SONG: <u>"Patience" by The Lumineers</u>

HIGHLIGHTED POSE/TRANSITION: Dead bug pose.

JOURNAL PROMPT: *Choose one something you are ready to let go of. Tear this page out of your journal and burn it.*

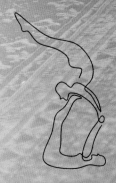

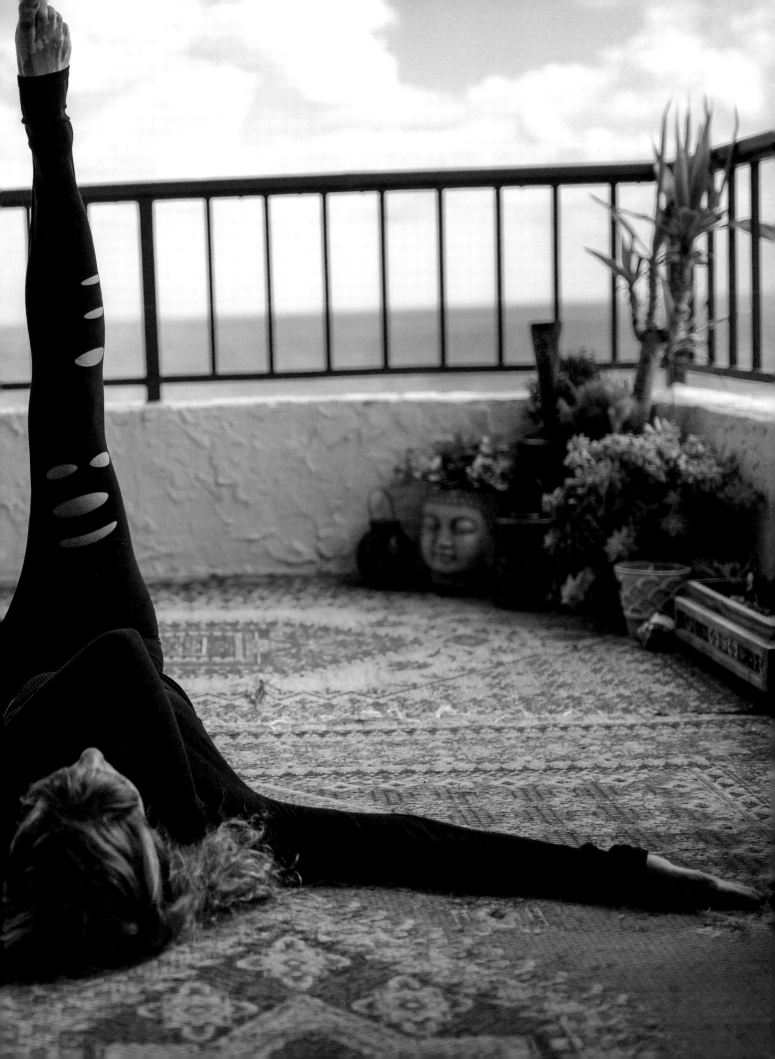

45. THEME: YOU ARE READY NOW

With challenging shapes, whether inverting or not, the intention coming in should be to break through thoughts like "I can't do that," "I'm not ready," or even "I'll never be able to do that." Try on "I am ready now" in the same way you would try on a shirt a friend is asking you to try on that maybe you don't see yourself in.

We all have a variety of excuses on hand when we don't feel ready for something! You may have thought or said, "I'll be ready when this pandemic is over, when I have more money, when tension in my relationship is resolved, when I process past trauma, when I'm living in my dream home, when my body is healed, when I lose another five pounds, when I am an expert in my industry, or when I…"

You are ready now!

When we arrive to this present moment with a deep sense of gratitude, we can hold space for what has been and our intention for this moment (and the future), and yet we can honor all we have done that has brought us to this space. We can continue to cultivate self-study and self-development and also break free of the shackles that create limiting beliefs.

Mantra practice: *I am enough. Breathe this in. Breathe this out. Repeat.*

You can achieve the benefits of an inversion practice in child's pose, in downward-facing dog, or anytime the legs and/or feet are above the heart. Legs-up-the-wall is a great one! When an inversion practice is called in class, you can access your variation for the moment. If it is safe for you to come into a headstand or forearm stand, and these shapes are new to you, please take care to practice at the wall, never jumping in. You know your body better than anyone, so take care to move into these challenging shapes attentively, with breath and trust.

A lot has been written and spoken about the sympathetic (fight-or-flight) and the parasympathetic (rest and digest) nervous systems. In the asana (pose) yoga practice, I often draw parallels between how we respond to challenge on the mat and how we respond to challenge off the mat. Sometimes our response is to freeze. I tend to freeze in extreme situations, a response triggered by psychological fear. When we understand the science behind why we are reacting and thinking the way we are, perhaps we can begin peeling back the layers to discover that we are more ready than we know.

VIDEO: <u>Know That You Are Ready Now</u>

PLAYLIST: <u>Say Something</u>

FEATURED SONG: <u>"Let It Be" by Kobor Gales</u>

HIGHLIGHTED POSES/TRANSITIONS: Headstand or forearm stand.

JOURNAL PROMPT: *Knowing you are ready now, what will you do with this beautiful life of yours?*

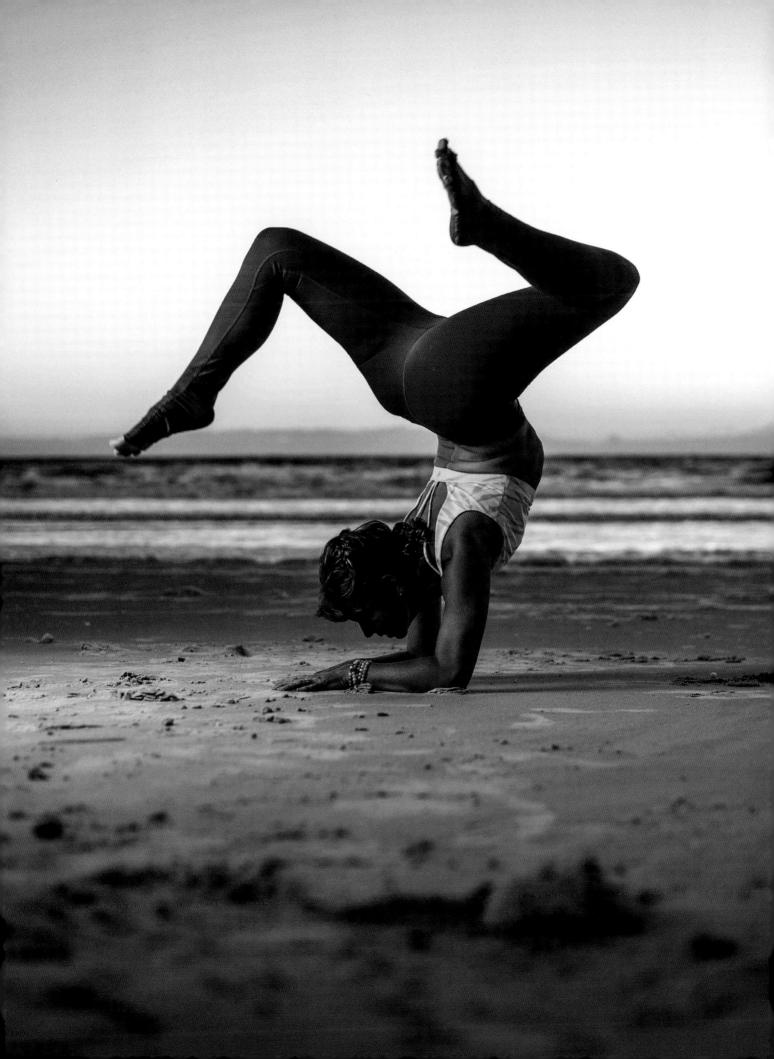

46. THEME: GYANA MUDRA

This is the beginning of a little mudra series. A mudra is a hand gesture or energy lock that helps you transform energy into more prana in your yoga practice. Gyana Mudra, or Chin Mudra, is known as the "Mudra of Knowledge" and is directly connected to the root chakra.

The root chakra connects to feeling grounded, secure, and stable.

Connect your index finger and thumb together like the OK symbol to bring together individual and universal consciousness. Here we connect to ourselves, to our loved ones, to those we know peripherally, and to those we have not met yet. We breathe with this mudra to tune into our collective consciousness, knowing that what unites us is greater than what divides us.

Attain true knowledge by realizing all the answers are already inside of you and in the natural intelligence of your body.

I like to find this mudra in a meditation seat. The palms could face up to connect to more receptivity or down to feel more grounded. I also like to flow with this mudra in a Vinyasa practice. My favorite shapes to embrace this mudra are triangle and peaceful warrior, where the top hand expresses the mudra, and warrior III, with the arms alongside the body and both hands expressing the mudra.

Gyana mudra is excellent for focus and concentration. It gives me the sense of connection and also the feeling that I'm holding on to something. Most of all, I feel a strong connection to myself. Sometimes I like to imagine people from all over the world practicing at the same moment, as well as all those who practiced before me. I find a tremendous peace honoring all the teachers before me who brought this practice, the mudras, and these teachings into existence. It's one of the most beautiful storytelling legacies, passed down for generations from 2700 BC.

VIDEO: <u>Gyana Mudra</u>
PLAYLIST: <u>Hope</u>
FEATURED SONG: <u>"Rays of Hope" by Oneke</u>

HIGHLIGHTED POSE/TRANSITION: Peaceful triangle with Gyana Mudra.

JOURNAL PROMPT: *What action will you take to connect to yourself? What action will you take to connect to others?*

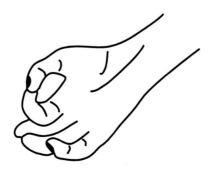

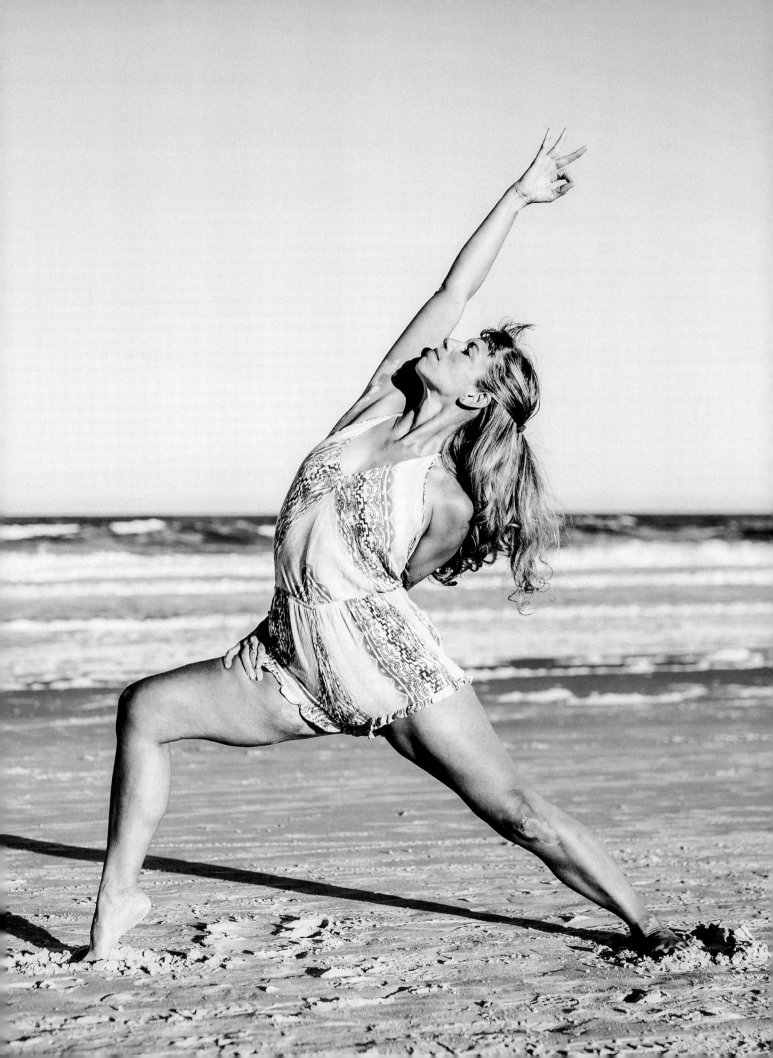

47. THEME: ANJALI MUDRA

This mudra may be the most popular or most practiced in yoga classes. You can find this hand gesture by joining the palms together. I tend to guide students to find Anjali Mudra, or prayer hands, sometimes at the beginning of class to set an intention, and always at the end of class. The invitation is to affirm or reaffirm our collective intention of the class's theme or any intention or dedication the students would like to set.

Practicing with Anjali Mudra generates feelings of love, peace, and compassion by expressing gratitude for all you possess. It is a simple and powerful gesture to intentionally bring peace into your life.

Breathe in "I am grateful for…" Breathe out: name what you are grateful for. Repeat. Breathe in stillness with this mudra or find movement with the mudra through twists and balances.

My favorite shapes to express this mudra are in a seated meditation, while chanting Om, Warrior I, Warrior III, chair, twisted chair, twisted high or low lunge, and yogi squat. I like to play with pressing left palm into right and right palm into left and feeling the energy of my intention between my palms. Sometimes I'll separate my palms ever so slightly and feel for that energy still residing there.

When we feel like we are in a space of scarcity or grasping, a gratitude practice can be very powerful to shift our mindset. Our gratitude practice can highlight the abundance we possess. Ultimately, this gratitude practice with the help of Anjali Mudra brings us to a space of peace within.

Intention setting with this mudra is one of the most powerful practices. I've planted many seeds here with each practice and I've witnessed how they manifest. I like to think of these intentions as putting a call out to the universe. Oftentimes my intention is love—love for myself, for my loved ones, for my students, for the strangers I pass on the street, for those I may never meet—I think of this intention setting as a devotional gesture so that I show up pure and present, mindful and aware, compassionate and receptive. My hope is this love has a beautiful ripple effect on all the lives I touch and those lives spread the love to the lives they touch and so on.

VIDEO: <u>Anjali Mudra</u>

PLAYLIST: <u>Gratitude</u>

FEATURED SONG: <u>"Lokah Samastah Sukino Bhavantu" by Jane Winther</u>

HIGHLIGHTED POSE/TRANSITION: Crescent lunge with prayer twist.

JOURNAL PROMPT: *What are you grateful for?*

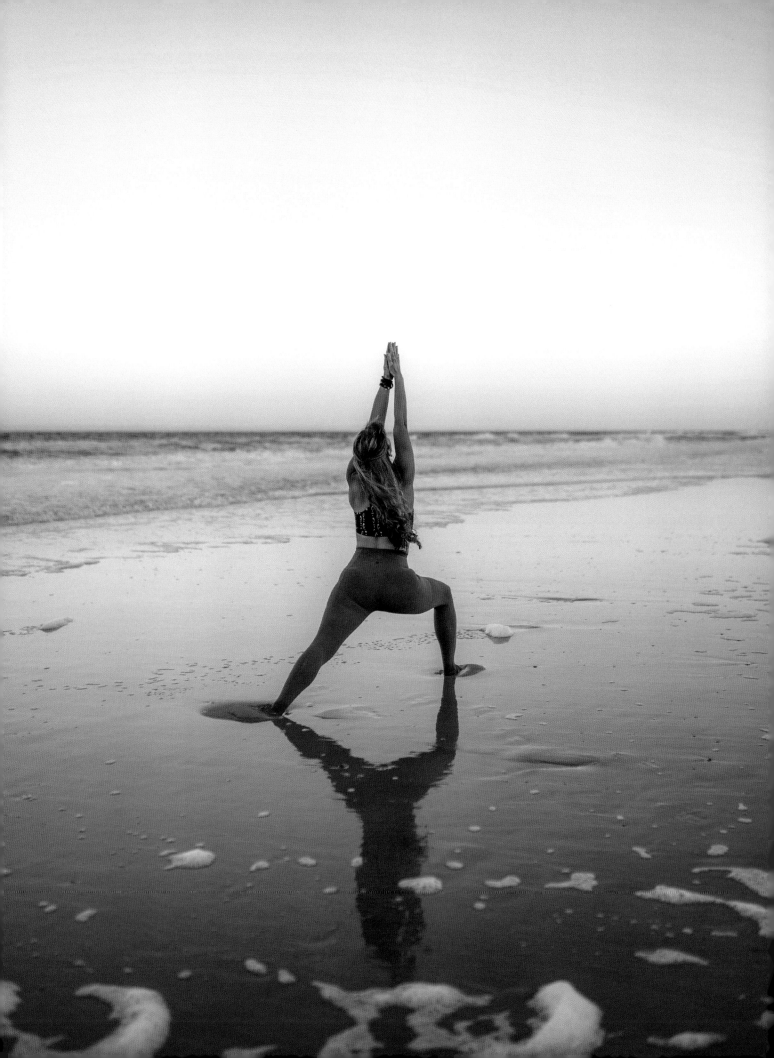

48. THEME: FEARLESS HEART MUDRA

Abahaya means "fearless," and hrdaya means "heart," "center or core of something," or "essence." This mudra, or symbolic gesture, helps strengthen a fearless connection to your heart's truth and grow your courage to follow that truth.

Bring your hands together in Anjali Mudra. Cross your right wrist over your left wrist in front of your sternum at the center of the chest, with the palms facing away from each other. Bring the backs of your hands together. Wrap your right index finger around the left index finger, then your right middle finger over your left, skip over the ring finger and wrap your right little finger over your left. Extend your ring fingers and thumbs out to each other to make a seal. Draw the mudra to the root of your heart, at the base of the sternum.

This mudra can increase the flow of energy in the heart, giving us courage to act from our fearless heart, and to let go of all that blinds us and binds us, to no longer be a hostage. It grounds scattered feelings and thoughts and brings us back to the heart's center. Having a fearless heart, to me, means loving fully, without qualifiers, listening to my heart's messages without my brain getting in the way, and pursuing my dreams with love as my driving intention.

What does having a fearless heart mean to you? As I meditate on this, to me, a fearless heart feels like a balance between strength and vulnerability. I recently saw a TED talk by Brené Brown about vulnerability. This talk struck many cords with me because I too love to be in control and yearn to have everything quantifiable. When we take into account fear and shame and cynicism and really all the learned behaviors we may adopt from trauma, it is no wonder how scarce it is to find those that are fully open, completely vulnerable, and free of expectation. I practice these qualities when I meet someone new as well as with loved ones.

When I worked in theatre there was a false closeness with fellow cast members. We're all thrust together for much of our days. And if we're lucky, we all get along. I've forged tremendous friendships this way, where we crack our hearts open and tell our deepest secrets to one another. Then, when the show closes, very often we seldom see each other again. "Life" takes over. After every show I did, I would mourn. I would mourn the loss of doing the show, the loss of the character I played and delved into so fully and completely, and the loss of the souls involved in the production that I'll likely only see on Facebook from this point forward. This cycle would repeat show after show from 2000 through 2019. It's a wonder I kept opening myself up to the loss. I suppose the connections made, even though they were fleeting, felt strong enough to carry me through. Our hearts are very resilient after all. I'd rather open my heart unabashedly than hide my heart for fear of getting hurt.

VIDEO: <u>Abhaya Hrdaya Mudra</u>
PLAYLIST: <u>The Water Lets You In</u>
FEATURED SONG: <u>"Forgive" by Trevor Hall, Luka Lesson</u>

HIGHLIGHTED POSE/TRANSITION: High Stance Pyramid with your heart cracked open.

JOURNAL PROMPT: *What does having a fearless heart mean to you?*

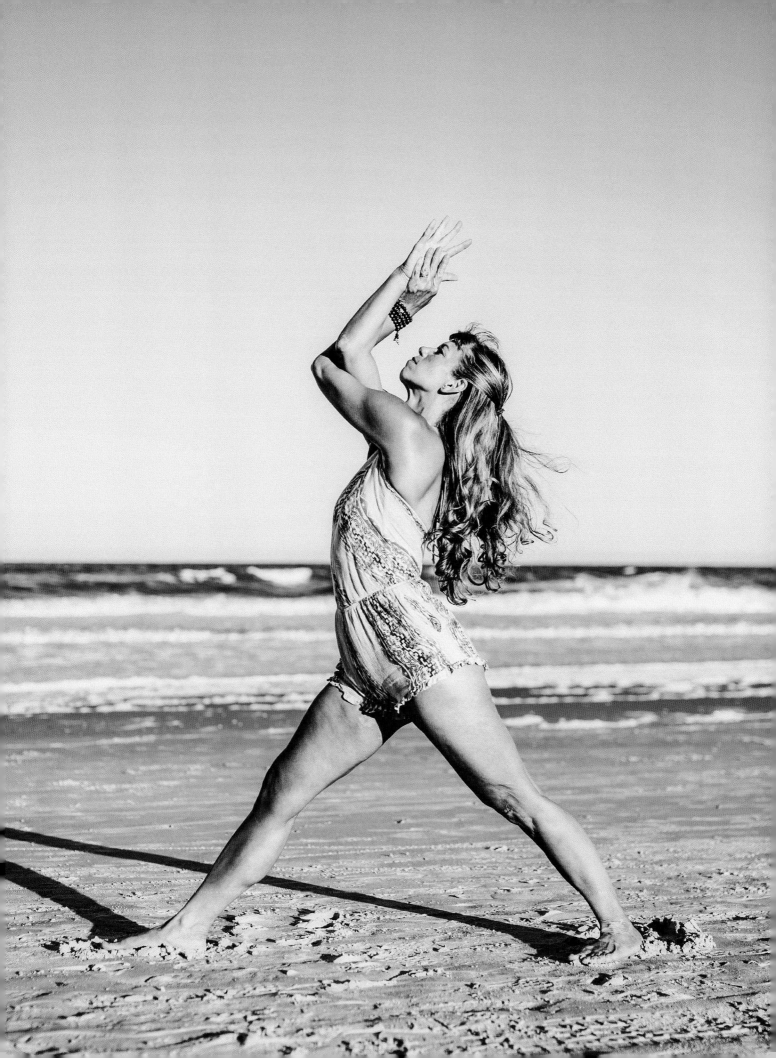

49. THEME: GANESHA MUDRA

Ganesha is a Hindu deity depicted as a richly adorned elephant meditating in the lotus position. He is both the remover of obstacles and responsible for placing certain obstacles in one's path in order to develop strength and resilience. The Ganesha mudra is therefore considered energetically strengthening, both physically and emotionally.

This gesture begins in Anjali Mudra. Start in a seated, comfortable position with your hands pressed together in prayer position at heart level. Keeping your palms together, swivel each hand so your fingertips point toward the opposite elbow, keeping your right palm facing your body. Bend all of your fingers on both hands into hooks. Slide your palms away from one another until your fingers hook together and lock.

Hold this pose for at least five minutes, or as long as you meditate. Chanting a Ganesh mantra, such as "Om Gam Ganapataye Namaha," can strengthen the power of this mudra.

My favorite shapes to express this mudra in are seated meditation or incorporating it into the sun salutations. Starting in Mountain Pose with Ganesha Mudra, carry the mudra up with you for volcano pose. Then break free the mudra as you spill down for forward fold. The same can be expressed through any lunge or warrior series: rise with the mudra in Warrior I, for example, and then break free to lower. This exploration of holding the obstacle and breaking free of it is freedom embodied!

As we explore the obstacles of the present moment, I invite you to examine which obstacles are self-made and which are outside of yourself. We as humans are tremendous storytellers, and we do a phenomenal job convincing ourselves of our current reality. So the invitation this week is to explore how obstacles show up in your life and your role in their existence.

We've all been there, in a sense, and have had the feeling of something or someone as an inhibitor. One of my favorite practices in these instances is asking, "What can I learn about myself here?" We can breathe through a tremendous amount when we remain curious.

VIDEO: <u>Ganesha Mudra</u>

PLAYLIST: <u>Hold On, Again</u>

FEATURED SONG: <u>"Inner Peace" by Beautiful Chorus</u>

HIGHLIGHTED POSE/TRANSITION: Bound extended side angle.

JOURNAL PROMPT: *What current obstacle do you have the power to remove?*

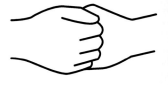

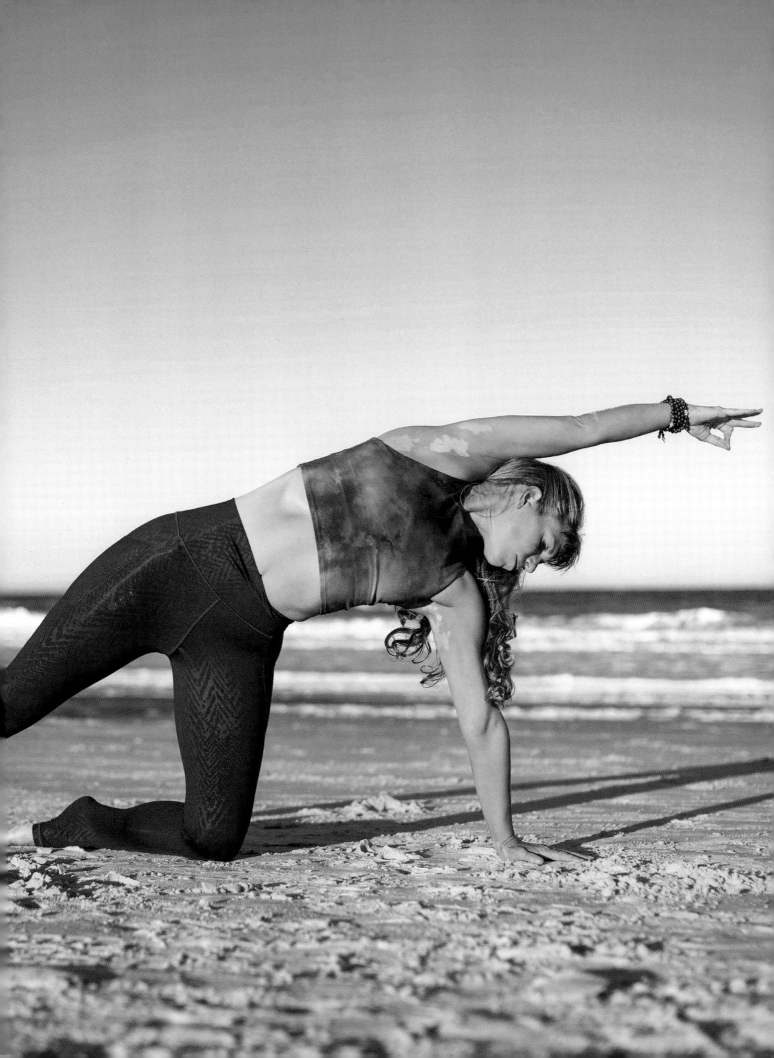

50. THEME: GARUDA MUDRA

Garuda Mudra is named after the eagle Vishnu—the lord of preservation—rides. It can help you cultivate the discipline you need to stick with your daily yoga practice when life gets busy or challenging. Garuda in Sanskrit means eagle. The symbol of an eagle makes me think of lightness and freedom.

This gesture is found by turning your hands so that the palms face up. Cross your right hand over your left, clasping your thumbs. Let the rest of the fingers of the hands stay extended, keeping the palms open.

Unlike most mudras, the Garuda Mudra uses the connection between both hands, locked together with the thumbs. This act brings balance between both sides of the body. The practice of Garuda Mudra is done with all the fingers stretched out, allowing them to be free. This gesture is said to also encourage you to let go and set yourself free. The practice of Garuda Mudra when done along with meditation cultivates a sense of control over the mind and a sense of orientation, just like the mighty eagle.

My favorite shapes to find this mudra are the same as with the Ganesha Mudra: seated meditation and incorporating it into sun salutations. Additionally, it feels quite lovely to find this mudra with eagle legs. It's a tricky balance when first playing with this variation, but if you feel confident in your eagle pose, it's a fun way to explore a different variation. When you feel steady in this variation, I invite you to shift your drishti (gaze) to your thumbs or even close your eyes.

My new morning ritual has brought me a lot of freedom. I now awake before the sunrise so I have time for all my Ayurveda rituals, meditation, journaling, reading, movement, and walking Bowery. This routine brings me much physical and mental freedom. My creativity is stimulated and I feel energized for the day. Carving this time out for myself has truly made me feel like I can soar in all I do!

VIDEO: <u>Garuda Mudra</u>

PLAYLIST: <u>The Garden</u>

FEATURED SONG: <u>"Flower of the Universe" by Sade</u>

HIGHLIGHTED POSE/TRANSITION: Eagle pose.

JOURNAL PROMPT: *What action can you take this week to bring you closer to freedom?*

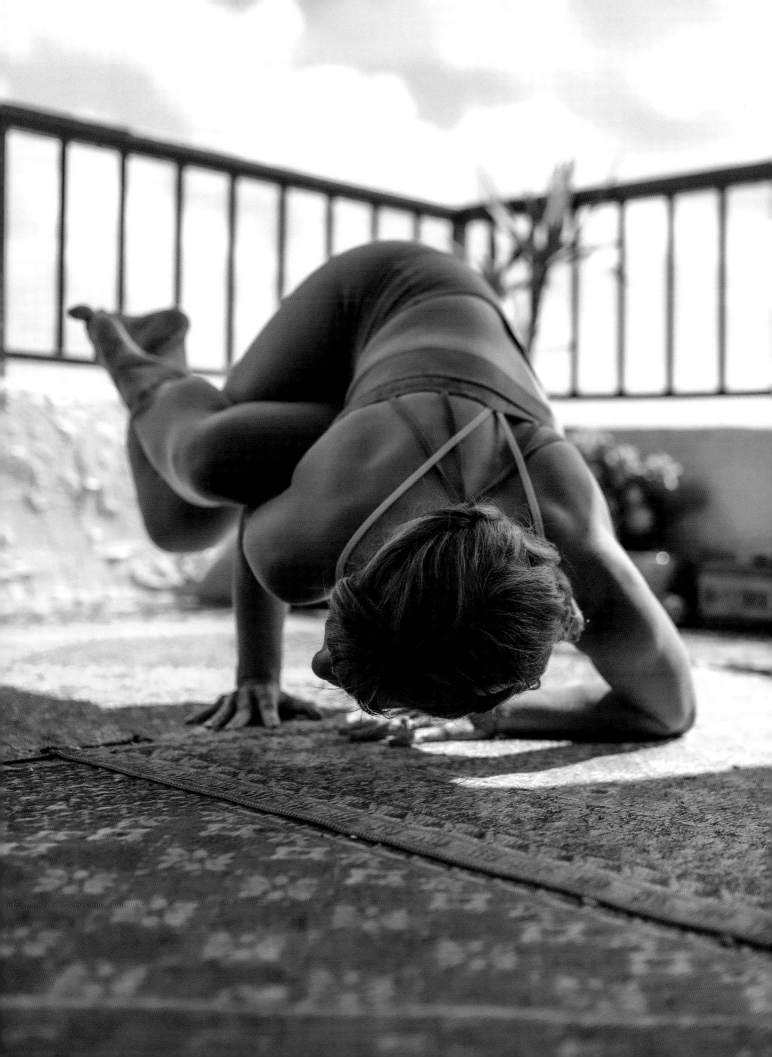

51. THEME: KALESVARA MUDRA

Kalesvara Mudra helps you take control of your mind. This mudra is dedicated to Kalesvaram (a synonym of Shiva), the Lord of Time. It helps us observe our character and contemplate our behavior. When you practice it consistently, you will observe reduced anxiety and better control over your thoughts and emotions. Kalesvara Mudra is also known to help in quitting addictions.

Put the pad of your middle fingers together. Touch the first two joints of your index fingers plus touch your thumbs. Curve your other fingers inward. End your thumbs in the direction of your chest. At the present extend out your elbows to the exterior. Breathe in and out gradually ten times. Then watch your breath and elongate the pause longer than the inhalation and exhalation. Focus on the habit you want to give up, or the change you want to create, and visualize it happening.

Kalesvara Mudra cools down the mind and therefore cools the flood of opinion. It also calms nervous feelings. As we become calmer, we will create more time and space between our thoughts. This will give us clarity and can potentially open us up to new perceptions of ourselves. In fact, Kalesvara Mudra is one of the best ways to make changes to your life because it opens you up to making changes to yourself, beginning with keeping your mind and body flexible. It can improve memory and concentration. You may even find yourself discovering unexpected solutions to conflicts you have been struggling with internally. You can carry these discoveries off the mat, allowing them to improve your health, your relationships, etc. The calmer your mind, the more clearly you will be able to think.

Remember that no mudra gives us instant results. You need to practice it daily for the recommended amounts of time. Mudras help channel the flow of energy in the body. They not only cleanse the body, they also remove toxic thoughts and ideas from the mind. If you are a person who struggles with a restless mind, if you find yourself constantly fending off unwanted thoughts, trying to deal with your anger, hatred, and irritation in a constructive way, or even struggling with addiction, Kalesvara Mudra can bring about a positive change. Before you attempt the mudra, you first need to focus on the traits you would like to change in yourself. Examine how you spend your time and seek out opportunities for increased mindfulness along the way. You will soon be surprised to discover how much you've changed!

Many of us have become more the human doing than the human being. I relish in multitasking and crossing things off my to-do list; it's one of my favorite pastimes. One area I try to avoid multitasking in is eating. I know very well that when I'm eating en route, watching something, reading, or writing emails, I'm not really tasting the food. The prana or the energy we consume is deeply felt when we multitask when eating. My recent practice has been pausing with the food in front of me and breathing in gratitude. I am grateful I have the opportunity to eat fresh and delicious foods at every meal. I give thanks to all those who played a role in harvesting the food so it is possible for me to eat. Then I take a bite and pay attention to the textures and tastes. It's not a true eating meditation at every meal; it's more of a mindfulness practice. This kind of awareness or concentration practice is akin to meditation. It is here that I savor "doing" less so I can experience more.

VIDEO: <u>Kalesvara Mudra</u>
PLAYLIST: <u>The Water Lets You In</u>
FEATURED SONG: <u>"The Course" by Ayla Nereo</u>

HIGHLIGHTED POSES/TRANSITIONS: Mindful movement Crescent Lunge into Warrior III.

JOURNAL PROMPT: *Choose one activity this week to resist multitasking in, or choose a task you've been procrastinating to do this week. Write down the activity, write down when you will do it, and make a note of any little steps you need to accomplish in order to complete it.*

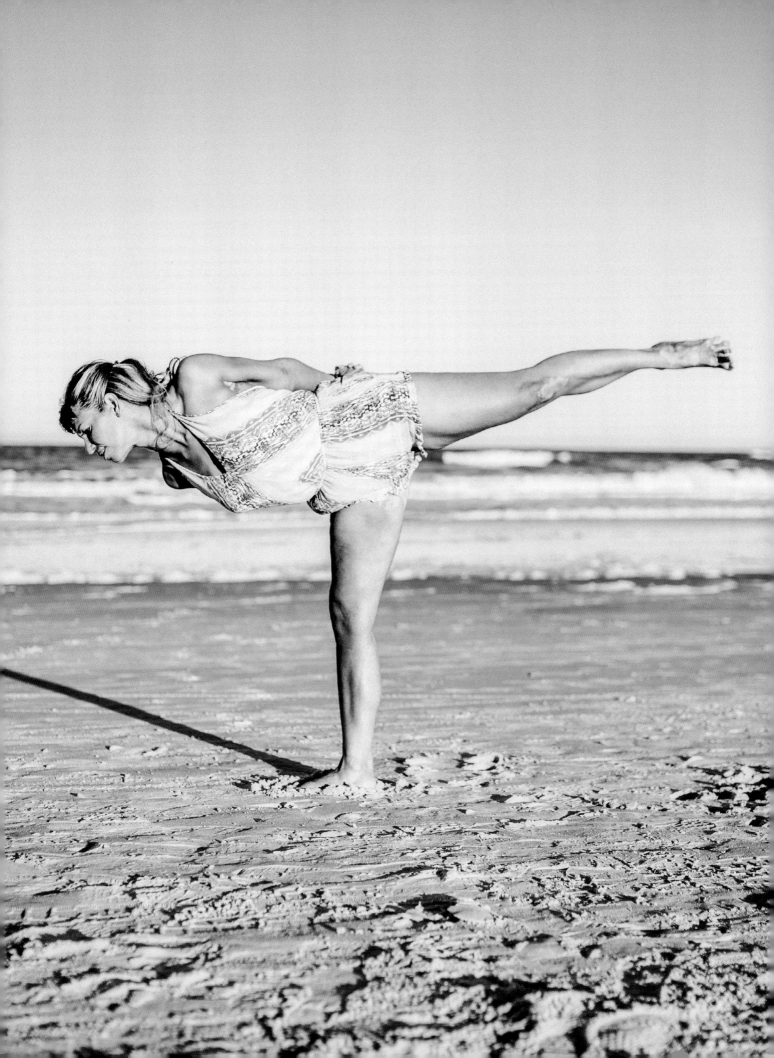

52. THEME: PRANA MUDRA

This mudra involves three fingers: the thumb, the ring finger, and the little finger. The Prana Mudra is considered one of the important mudras because of its benefits. As the name suggests, it enhances the vital energy in the body.

The Prana Mudra is simple to do. Just join the tips of the little finger, the ring finger, and the thumb together, with the other two fingers relaxed and positioned away from the joint. While practicing the mudra, you may sit in a comfortable position. Rest both hands on your knees and then fold the fingers into the mudra. While practicing it, give slight attention to your breathing patterns and allow the soothing effects of refreshed energy to calm your body and mind.

Tune in to your life force, your energy, how you are expending your energy and, without judgment, observe how you feel.

Of the five fingers, our thumb represents agni (fire), the little finger represents jala (water), and the ring finger represents prithvi (earth).

The benefits of practicing the Prana Mudra and the ease with which you can practice it show that this is the best practice that you can incorporate into your daily routine.

Expressing your prana and being mindful of your own prana is the essence of my mission statement. I am here to help guide you to shine your light both on and off the mat. Through these themes, these practices, and these journal prompts there are many portals into the self to explore. Through this Svadhyaya (self-study) we may begin to peel the layers of the onion to reveal your truest and purest self. It's a lifelong journey I am committed to and I hope you can feel the impact of your light energy now that you've arrived at week fifty-two. I am proud of you for arriving at this point on your path. You can rinse and repeat this series every year. As you continue to grow and change, each timely and timeless theme will strike you in different ways. I'm excited to be a part of your journey. This is the end and it is also the beginning.

VIDEO: <u>Prana Mudra</u>

PLAYLIST: <u>Someday</u>

FEATURED SONG: <u>"Here, Right Now" by Joshua Radin</u>

HIGHLIGHTED POSE/TRANSITION: Fierce Crescent Pose with Prana Mudra.

JOURNAL PROMPT: *How will you show up in a way that lets your light shine today, this week, and onward?*

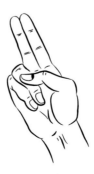

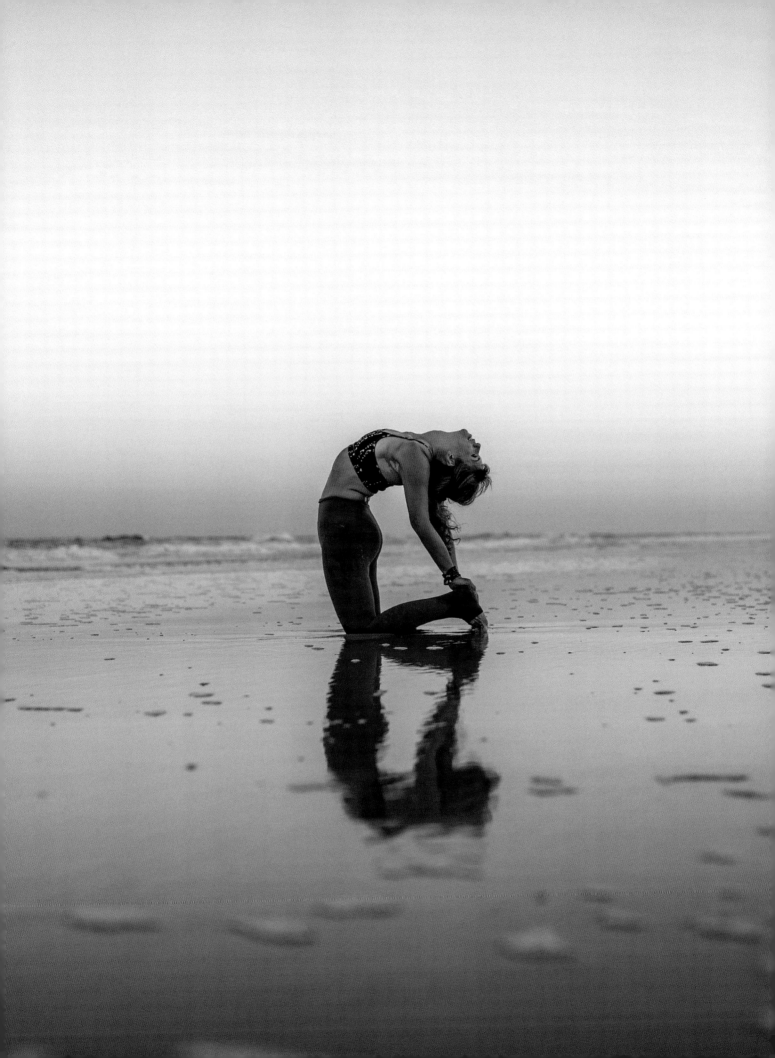

EPILOGUE

I began writing this book seven weeks before the pandemic, before I had space
(Read: time in my schedule) to create videos, and here are the initial seeds of this book.

1. THEME: "TAKE CARE OF YOUR BODY. IT'S THE ONLY PLACE YOU HAVE TO LIVE." —JIM ROHN

The two most important days in your life are the day you are born and the day you find out why.

—Mark Twain

Hurricane Dorian is the first hurricane I've lived through. With all the yoga studio closures and being told to stay inside, all I could do was stay home and watch the news. I didn't know if this hurricane would take everything from us, and the stress of the unknown materialized in a horrible stomach pain I'd never experienced before.

Thankfully the hurricane did not end up hitting our little beach town, but the pain in my stomach remained. For my entire life, I've always shown up to my commitments without fail, but it was getting increasingly challenging to teach. My stomach was seriously inflamed, and I was finding myself needing to sit down and simply talk through the sequence, unable to demonstrate or walk around at all. Finally I decided to go to urgent care, where the doctor immediately told me I needed to go to the ER. Now I was scared! They ran a bunch of tests and could not determine why I was having so much pain. After eight hours, they sent me home with a prescription for painkillers and no answers. I was referred to a GI doctor, who recommended an upper endoscopy and determined I had gastritis and inflammation of the stomach. He prescribed medicine to reduce the inflammation.

All of this is to say that yoga is a practice. There are events in our lives that challenge us to remember our breath and what we are taking in that is helpful versus harmful. I am acutely aware now that the intake of news surrounding all these unknowns—the anticipation, the anxiety surrounding the "what if"—isn't healthy for anyone. Finding the balance between being informed and being completely overcome with anxiety is a balance only you can find for yourself.

It all begins with a conscious awareness of how the mind plays a tremendous role in our physical health and then taking an active part to take care of both the mind and the body with the same respect.

PLAYLIST: <u>Opening</u>
FEATURED SONG: "<u>The Call</u>" by <u>Regina Spektor</u>

HIGHLIGHTED POSES/TRANSITIONS: Child's pose. Mindful movements with heightened awareness of mind–body connection and taking rest when the mind or the body calls for it.

JOURNAL PROMPT: *What is a recent challenge, whether physically, mentally, or emotionally, that you overcame? How did you overcome this challenge?*

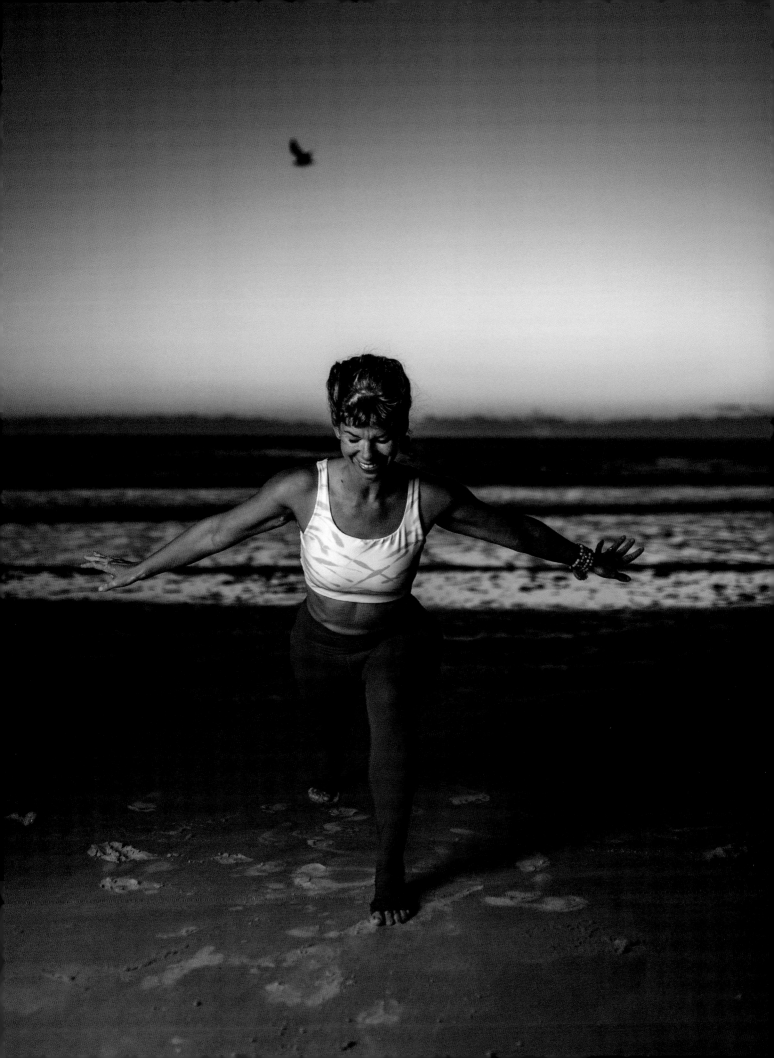

2. THEME: SLOWING DOWN

I try to fill my days with as much as I can. I love crossing things off my to-do list. I sometimes forget to be a human being, not a human doing. I was running late to teach this week. And I was reminded to slow down by a kind, yet authoritative police officer when he pulled me over. In this age of multitasking and technology, we may find ourselves driving while eating, while also talking on the phone, and thinking about what we are supposed to do next. Perhaps it's not entirely realistic in a modern world to simply do one thing at a time and never find ourselves running late. However, we can pay more attention to when it's actually necessary to run around and when there are opportunities to slow down.

Do you find that you're always that person who is apologizing for being late? Perhaps it's time to acknowledge that you can reexamine your priorities. Often, we can more effectively show up when we show up slowly, with intention, in order to be more present once we've arrived.

When I lived in NYC and LA, I always felt like I was running behind. Part of that was because of "mass transit" and "traffic," respectively. But I was also compulsively trying to fit too much into any given day and therefore I didn't give myself windows between appointments for potential red lights, let alone mindful meals. So it's probably no coincidence that of all the unique themes I've come up with over the year, this is the only one that repeats.

I will say I come by my attitude quite honestly. Both my parents are "retired," and yet when I call them, they've both said on multiple occasions, "I don't know how I was able to get anything done while I was working." I suppose it is a natural inclination for some of us to fill the hours, minutes, and nanoseconds given to us.

As I write this, I currently have carved two full days off! This is a huge deal for me as, for most of my adult life, I have made it a point to work every day. Part of that comes from a freelancer mentality of saying yes to all of the work because you don't know when it will stop, and I think the other part is a deeply seeded belief of attaching my self-worth to how much I'm doing. I know that was true in LA and NYC. Now in Vero Beach, I'm rounding the bend to notice how I can actually slow down in a way that feels fulfilling to me. On the mat, that could look like the slowest transition from half-moon pose to goddess pose, or simply lingering in a shape that feels really good. Off the mat, I'm enjoying carving time out for slow and mindful meals. I take a beat before I eat, look at the food, and express gratitude. I try to limit distraction so I can take mindful bites and breathe into embracing food as medicine.

PLAYLIST: <u>Easy Tiger</u>

FEATURED SONG: <u>"Let It Go" by Colin & Caroline</u>

HIGHLIGHTED POSES/TRANSITIONS: Thread the needle, walking
meditation from downward-facing dog to the top of the mat.

JOURNAL PROMPT: *What's one way you can slow down? What's one activity you can do mindfully?*

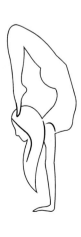

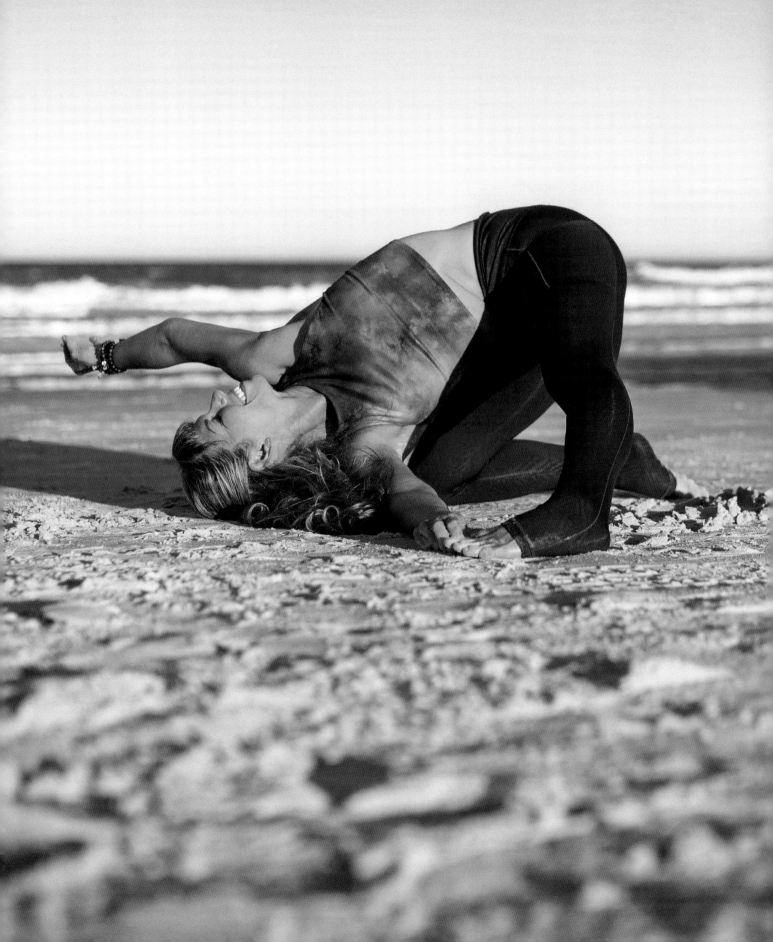

3. THEME: SELF-EMPOWERMENT

Claiming your power to accept challenges, claiming your power to take rest, and claiming your power to modify when needed happens on the mat with a challenging sequence with a lot of core exercises, and happens off the mat when we are challenged in relationships or conversations, or dealing with changes when things don't go as we planned. The invitation is to choose a mantra for your practice. Maybe choose a mantra you love or choose a new one. If you're looking for a new one, think of a quality you'd like to embody here and now—the first word that comes to mind. Perhaps silently repeat that word to yourself again and again, or make it an affirmation by adding the words "I am" in front of it. For example, "I am empowered." Repeat this mantra for the duration of practice or whenever you think of it.

I'll share a secret with you. Sometimes I trace my mantra or affirmation with my finger at the top of the mat. I pretend my finger is a paintbrush, a marker, or a fine-tipped pen, and I write my mantra out on my mat in cursive or in block letters. I visualize the mantra and it serves as a reminder to turn inward. With every thought that arises, I can see the mantra, catching me just as I am and encouraging me along.

Now carry this mantra with you off the mat and repeat it to yourself in those times you need to feel empowered.

PLAYLIST: <u>Patience</u>
FEATURED SONG: <u>"Lokah samastah sukhino bhavantu" by Jane Winther</u>

HIGHLIGHTED POSES/TRANSITIONS: Chair Pose, Fierce Crescent Lunge into Warrior III.

JOURNAL PROMPT: *Write down your mantra again and again until it sinks in.*

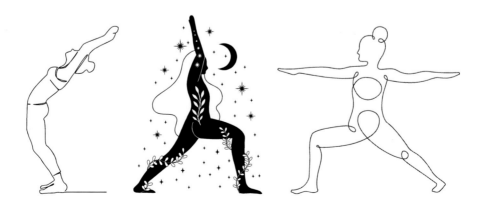

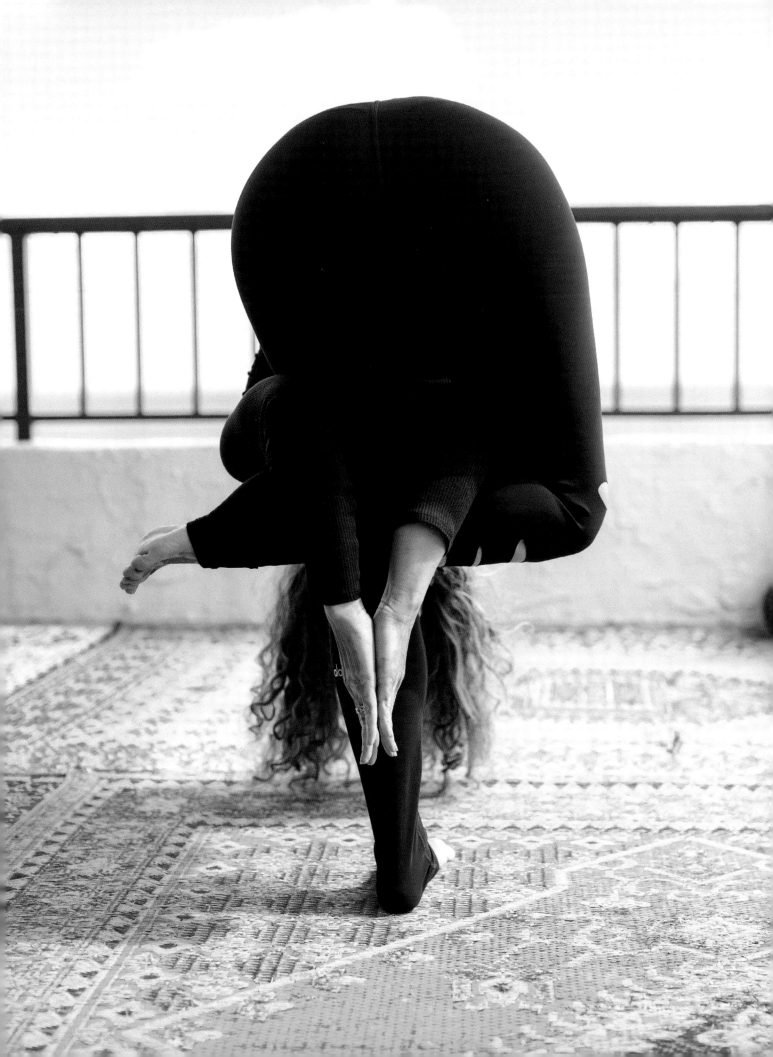

4. THEME: SELF-INQUIRY SURROUNDING YOUR TRIGGERS

Between stimulus and response there is a space. In that space is our power to choose our response. In our response, lies our growth and our freedom.

—Viktor E. Frankl

I am inspired to invite you to meditate, examine, and observe your triggers as I believe we all have triggers that catch us off guard, initiate an emotional response, and shift us to a fear-based reaction. Take this practice to recognize your triggers without judgment and see them from a place of compassion. Notice how you feel when you breathe into that space.

This is an opportunity to take yoga off the mat. Nothing requires a response right away. Now that you've cultivated an awareness of your triggers, you are empowered to rewrite your story. Breathe for sixteen counts and see how you feel now. Approach these moments as a chance to practice curiosity: how can this help me grow? Come from a place of ever evolving and always learning, and respond from love.

I don't mind sharing with you that one of my big triggers is feeling like my time is being wasted. This can happen when someone is late to an appointment, or when a meeting is taking longer than I think it should, when an event is not what I expected, or when I find myself stuck in traffic, or delayed in some way out of my control. Yep, I've spent a lot of time in these situations, I've spent a lot of time thinking about them, and, of course, recounting them to my loved ones. One consistent part of all of these situations where I feel like my time is being wasted is my feeling that it's out of my control. To me this is equal parts frustrating and liberating. Of course, the frustrating part is that it's out of my control. That's pretty self-explanatory. But the liberating part is also that it's out of my control. You can see how this internal battle can happen, right? I'm still working on this one, but I've come a long way.

One of the best ways I've come to approach this one is by asking myself, "What can I learn here?" When I greet frustration with curiosity, it changes my frame of mind. When someone is late to an appointment, it helps me to use it as an opportunity to catch up on email or to take mindful breaths. I try to remember these things aren't personal attacks (even though they feel that way sometimes) and that they're not happening to me, but happening for me.

PLAYLIST: <u>First Impressions</u>

FEATURED SONGS: <u>"Limitations" by East Forest</u>; <u>"Be Here Now" by Ray LaMontagne</u>

HIGHLIGHTED POSES/TRANSITIONS: Equal-parts breath—four-count inhale, four-count hold, four-count exhale, and four-count hold; Standing half-moon pose with hand bind; Warrior III with Yogi Mudra.

JOURNAL PROMPT: *Name one trigger you'd like to let go of. You can tear this page out of your journal and set it on fire.*

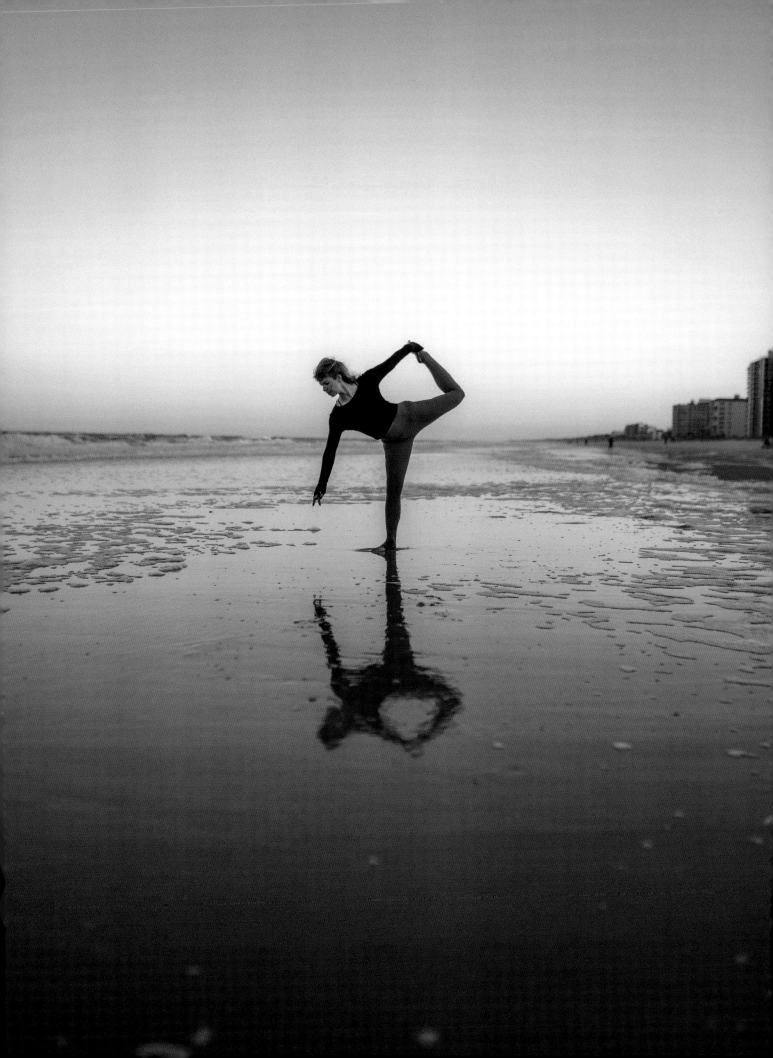

5. THEME: HEALING

Read from *Journey to the Heart* by Melody Beattie —

February 25: Learn to Help Heal Yourself

have been on the healing journey for the last 20 years. The journey to healing—I have found—has similar emotions to the grief journey: denial, acceptance, rage, impatience…and sometimes all of the emotions at once.

Somehow—out of nowhere—last week I awoke with a sense of peace surrounding my pain. Nothing had changed, however I felt an awakening that if nothing will change, I now feel ready to accept things as they are.

After many months away from *Journey to the Heart* by Melody Beattie, I felt pulled to read today's entry and found chills when I read the title: "Learn to Help Heal Yourself."

I was journaling a couple days ago, guided by Anthony DiFiglio. The prompt was "What do you know to be true?" My initial response was in the realm of "I'm a healer." He then led us through a handful of prompts where we questioned our beliefs, the container we have surrounding what we are willing to question. Then he circled back around to, "What do you know to be true?" My response in the end was in the realm of "I have a body." One of my fellow yoga teacher trainees shared her identification as a person with an autoimmune disease and her questioning now whether that is true. This hit me at the core.

I've struggled with this assigned label for more than twenty years now and have been labeling myself in the same way. I look at my skin and I think about my autoimmune disease. I look at other people's skin and I think about it as well. I'm not saying it monopolizes all of my thoughts, but I do think of it frequently. I have asked myself the question over and over, "What did I do to bring this on?" No one knows. My vitiligo may be my biggest teacher. This very superficial and cosmetically (im)perfect part of me appears through my eyes and in my reflection every day. I'm beginning to shift my healing practices from the inside out.

PLAYLIST: <u>Hope</u>
FEATURED SONG: <u>"Rays of Hope" by Oneke</u>

HIGHLIGHTED POSES/TRANSITIONS: Dead bug—shake off all the pain from your limbs and then let your arms and legs droop like they are in a jello mold: effortless, weightless, and without gravity.

JOURNAL PROMPT: *What healing practices are nonnegotiable for you?*

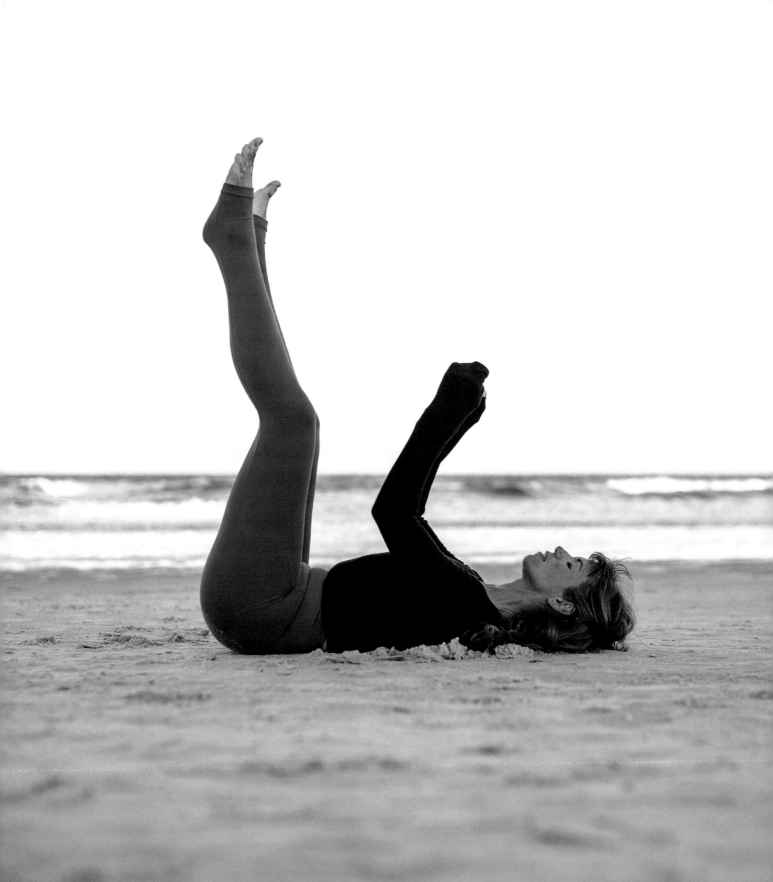

6. THEME: PRANAYAMA/ BREATH PRACTICE INSPIRED BY TAO PORCHON-LYNCH

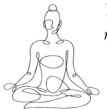

When I wake up in the morning, I know that it's going to be the best day of my life. I never think about what I can't do. Make sure positive thoughts are the first ones you think in the morning. And never procrastinate.

—Tao Porchon-Lynch

Tao Porchon-Lynch was the oldest yoga instructor in the world at 101 years young. She passed away a couple weeks ago. When asked what she attributed her long and healthy life to, she said the pranayama practice/the breath practice. With the focus on the breath being paramount to the asana practice/the poses we take, we are able to heal and nourish the body and mind. The invitation is to begin with a pranayama and centering practice. If and when you are craving movement, start slowly and keep the breath at the forefront.

Practice observing the breath and if you find the breath becomes shallow or you're holding your breath, please find a modification to the shape, slow down/speed up, find where challenge or rest are more apropos for you in each moment. Take this practice with you off the mat. Notice what happens to the breath when you're driving, when you're having an argument, when you're running late to an appointment. The simple act of simply observing the breath can shift the way you experience life. Guiding yourself to slow the breath down can certainly guide you closer to peace.

When I originally wrote this entry and planned and taught this class, we were openly breathing in close proximity to one another. That came to a halt in the early weeks of the pandemic. The studios eventually reopened, but I feel like I've been holding my breath ever since. I used to love guiding pranayama or breath practice, particularly in restorative or Yin practices. In all of my classes, I would guide a collective breath to begin and close practice. "Inhale your intention through the nose, exhale it out the mouth." Somehow with an airborne pandemic on our hands, a deep exhale out the mouth with sound hardly felt appropriate. Nor did any guided breath! In fact, in a weird, subconscious way, I've felt like I've tried to pretend that we don't need to breathe at all in an effort to make everyone feel more comfortable that we're all breathing in this enclosed space. It's been terribly maddening indeed!

I am certainly ready for that deep audible exhale! I read somewhere that our turtle friends breathe just four breaths per minute. Just four! It may be why they live so long. I think about that when I catch myself holding my breath or breathing quickly. I want to be here for as many days as I can. I aspire to be 101 years young.

PLAYLIST: <u>Opening</u>
FEATURED SONG: <u>"Stacks" by Bon Iver</u>

HIGHLIGHTED POSES/TRANSITIONS: Flow in Sun B. First build each shape and then take one flowing breath per movement. Flow in Crescent Lunge, Warrior II, Peaceful Warrior, Extended Side Angle, Peaceful Triangle, and Low Lunge open twist with option for Side Plank—Vinyasa.

JOURNAL PROMPT: *What is one activity you can do today to feel young?*

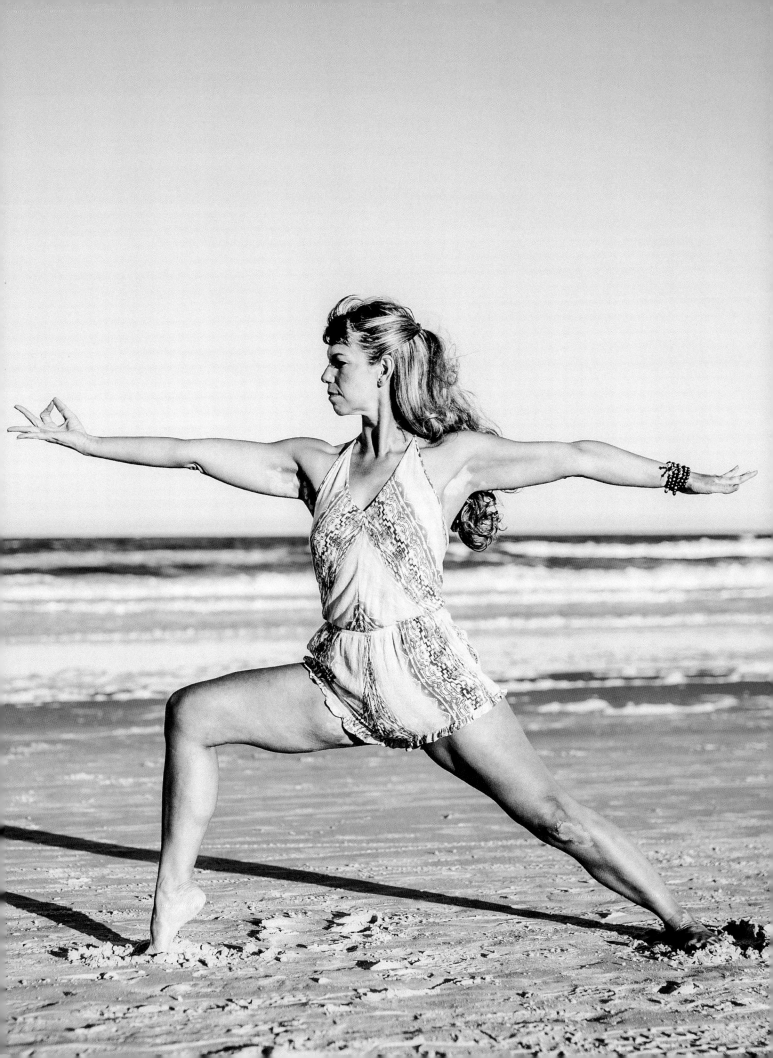

7. THEME: THE SUPER MOON

Agorgeous moon greeted me each evening and morning early this week, which is what inspired this sequence. The moon's energy has a reputation for making people crazy—especially combined with mercury in retrograde and the coronavirus to boot! Just like a lot of things where you can see different ways to interpret or respond to an event, this is true here. I invite you to embrace moon energy to inspire, energize, and spark creativity in you. Let the moonlight nourish and nurture you. And let the seeds of your intention harvest in the moonlight. Hydrate, wash your hands, and don't watch the news.

I remember this class very vividly. It was in fact the last week before the studios closed, before many businesses closed. I think of my friends in NYC and LA still under a shutdown in many ways. I am witness to the depression that has washed over much of this world during this time. The restriction of activity and touch just about crushes the human soul.

In this last super moon–inspired class, we were still mat to mat, I was still giving hands-on assists, we were still borrowing props, we were still hugging and gesturing with a gentle touch to the arm. On the other side of this, I have not hugged my mom in a year. The fear propagated by the media has left many of us very much further than six feet apart from our loved ones.

I don't have the answers. I observe with curiosity and try my best not to get pulled down the rabbit hole of fear-based emotions.

I'm excited that one of the studios where I teach, Rhythm & Soul, is implementing assist cards. One side says yes and the other side says no. Students can begin to express if they are ready to receive hands-on assists again. I know some preferred not to be touched before the pandemic, and my hope is we can build a culture in the yoga community that is more aware of everyone's comfort level. This, to me, is moon, maternal and nurturing energy. My hope is to provide tools where we can look at any given situation and ask, "What can this teach me?" I have learned, unlearned, and relearned so much in this past year. Some of the teachings have been uncomfortable and have left me asking, "What is true?" I invite you to embody your role as a truth seeker for yourself, in your relationships, and in your role in this world.

PLAYLIST: <u>Patience</u>

FEATURED SONG: <u>"Because" by the Beatles</u>

HIGHLIGHTED POSE/TRANSITION: Half-moon pose on your
back with a knee down and then on one foot.

JOURNAL PROMPT: *Write down one challenge. Rephrase this challenge in a way that inspires
you. Take action: allow this mindset shift to energize and spark creativity in you.*

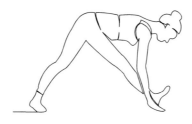

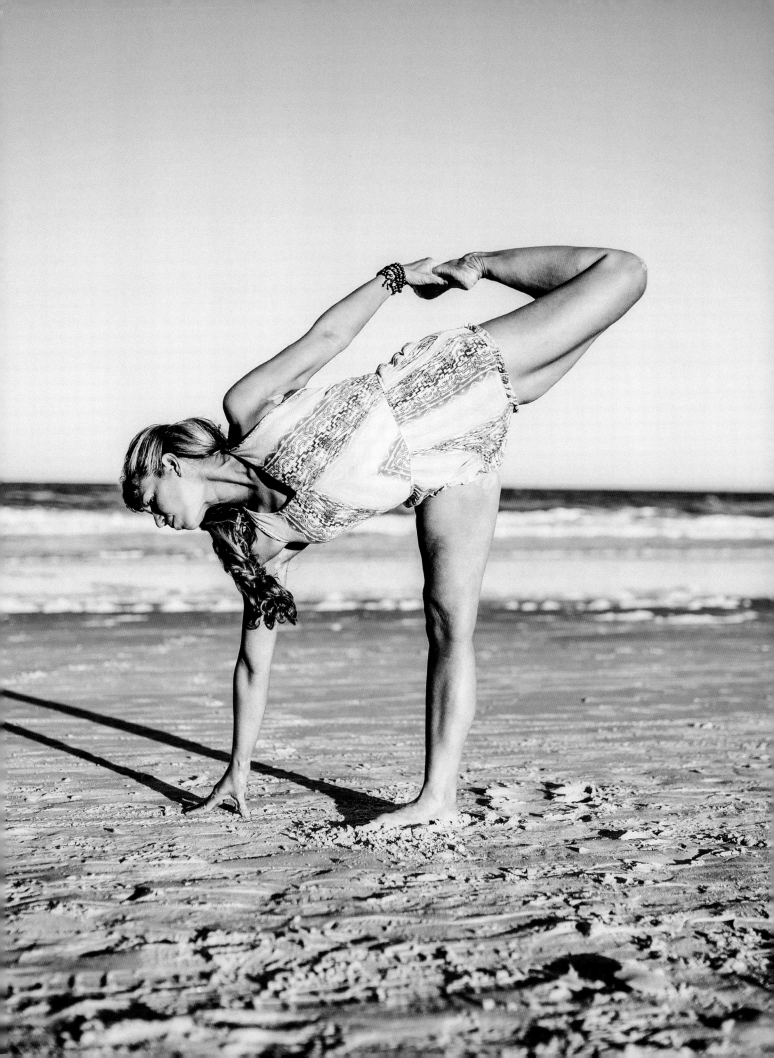

CONGRATULATIONS ON COMPLETING THIS YEARLONG SERIES. Notice for yourself what has changed, what has remained the same. I often regard this practice like peeling the layers of the emotional body like an onion—it takes time and chances are there will be tears. Sometimes you may be called to sit with these feelings, move through these emotions or stretch your perspective of your capacity to do hard things.

You are welcome to repeat this series year after year in the order I wrote this book or choose the theme that resonates for you in the moment. Go back and read your previous journal responses and add on year after year. May these timely and timeless themes serve you exactly where you are in this moment…and then this moment…and, yes, this moment too…

"When all is said and done, we're all just walking each other home."

—Ram Dass

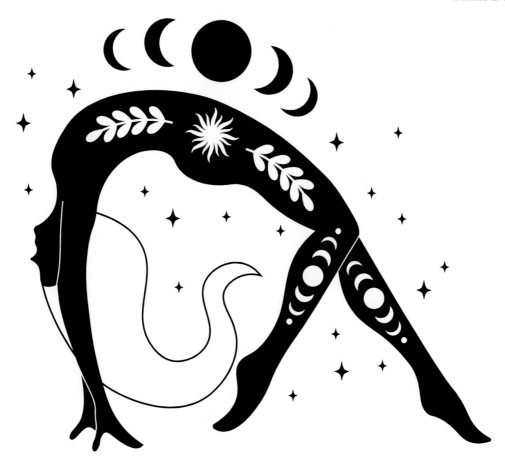

ACKNOWLEDGMENTS

am here because of my family, my friends, my teachers, my students and the experiences along the way that guided me.

To Brandon, who encouraged me to write my stories down, to become a yoga instructor, and to stay creative.

To my mom, who taught me to follow through with what I say I will do and to break the rules every now and then.

To my dad, who stands on his head and does crossword puzzles every day. His wit and thirst for knowledge inspire me.

To my grandfather Stephen, the original storyteller from my childhood who inspired me to use my voice in a way that is true.

To my stepmom, who taught me about Tiffany's etiquette and how to dress for the occasion.

To my teachers at Pure Yoga West: Kiley Holiday, Rebecca Hajek, Scott Harig, Domenic Savino, Dana Slamp, Miles Borrero, Lauren Taus; Jivamukti Yoga: Austin Sanderson; Surya Yoga Academy: Justin Randolph, Christina Hart, Angela Rauscher; The Yoga Room: Serena Tom, Wesley Collier.

Yoga retreats with Cortney Ostrosky at Blue Spirit (Costa Rica); Kiley Holiday and Amanda Murdock at Cap Maison (St. Lucia); Studio Bamboo/Ann Richardson Stevens (Maya Tulum); Kat Fowler at Kripalu (The Berkshires); Courtney Common and Alexandra Ann at Coco B Wellness (Isla Mujeres, Mexico).

Yoga teacher training with Amazing Yoga (Karen and Sean Conley), Flor Yoga (Sarah and Tomas Marsh, May Lane, Dr. Melanie Ann Llanes, and Autumn Perez) and Authentic Movements (Steph Gongora, Erin Kelly, and Bianca Scalise with Sean Michael Imler, Mr. Kim House, Dr. Dheepa Sundaram, Jenni Rawlings, Davina Davidson, Dr. Zac Cupples, Sam Vetrano, Dr. Ben House and Anthony Difliglio).

To my home studios and clubs over this past year: A Healthier Me, Good Life Fitness, Intergenerational Recreation Center, Level Yoga, Oak Harbor, Quail Valley, Rhythm & Soul, Spark of Divine, and Windsor—to the staff, my fellow teachers, and all the students who attend yoga classes here, thank you for showing up, for breathing, and for practicing.

Photography by the beautiful souls behind Light Wave Photography: Shazia Bashir and Jeff Tong.

Hair color, cut and style by Austin at BoHo House Salon. The only time I'm happy to sit for four hours is in your chair whilst you work your magic!

Book editing by Matt Popham. Book consulting by Janna Hockenjos. Your guidance to my meanderings has brought shape and clarity to each entry.

And, of course, thanks to Bowery, my yogi pup. I love you, buddy. Thanks for being by my side for my daily practice.

VERONIQUE ORY
Yoga Instructor

Originally from Montreal, Quebec, I'm a French-Canadian girl who loves the arts, yoga, coffee and finding adventure! I studied Theatre at Russell Sage College in Troy, NY. My theatre mentor guided me to move to Los Angeles to pursue film and TV. I acted in independent films, but missed my love of theatre. I formed my own non-profit theatre company, Athena Theatre, producing published TONY and Pulitzer Award Winning revival plays. I produced published and new plays in both LA and NYC for seventeen years. My love of the arts and storytelling was incredibly stressful because of the heightened emotions in the industry. I discovered yoga as a way to calm the mind and feel good in the body. I fell in love with the connection of storytelling and creative movement.

Currently based in Vero Beach, FL and a RYT (Registered Yoga Teacher with Yoga Alliance) 500 Yoga Instructor. I find inspiration off of the mat for unique and creative yoga teachings at each class. Every class is tailored to the setting, students and by an inspirational theme. I strive to empower and inspire my students to shine their light. I offer precise alignment cues as well as modifications to journey through class while mending an injury or expressing a more advanced practice. I love the use of descriptive words to guide practice and I also tune in to when to be silent, allowing space for each student to simply breathe.

I am mostly known for my smile;) I love to laugh! I am passionate, empathetic and love storytelling! I'm also adventurous and seek out travel and discovering new places. I get excited about active outings as well such as flying trapeze, rock climbing, high ropes courses and I did go sky diving once—once was enough! :) I am drawn to challenges and enjoy arm balances and going upside down in my yoga practice as well as exploring creative movement.

Certifications and Qualifications:

- Yoga Alliance Registered Yoga Teacher 100 hours with Amazing Yoga at Blue Spirit in Nosara, Costa Rica

- Yoga Alliance Registered Yoga Alliance Experienced 200 hours with Flor Yoga in Jersey City, NJ

- Yoga Alliance YACEP, Yoga Alliance Continuing Education Provider

- Yoga Alliance Registered Yoga Teacher 500 hours in Hatha, Vinyasa and Restorative with Authentic Movements

- A Journey into Yin with Travis Eliot

- 200 hours in Hatha, Vinyasa and Restorative with Authentic Movements

- 40+ hours in techniques, trainings and practice, teaching methodology, anatomy & physiology, yoga philosophy, lifestyle and ethics with Yoga Alliance, Pure Yoga in NYC, Kat Fowler, Ann Richardson + countless podcasts and webinars

I love serving the world by giving each person space to express themselves in a way where their light can radiate and shine for all to see. I believe I unlock physical and emotional blockages through my yoga teachings. I take great care in guiding each student on a path that is balanced between effort and ease—where they can embrace challenge while still feeling supported; ever evolving, ever growing!

The things I am most passionate about in life are wellness, mindfulness, traveling, teaching, family, friends and being the change I wish to see in the world! I'm passionate about continually challenging my beliefs, continuing to practice self-study, read and accrue new knowledge. I am passionate about recycling and limiting single use containers/bottles, not using straws and taking care of this environment.

When I'm not busy teaching you can find me practicing yoga with my dog, Bowery, or reading.

www.YogaWithVeronique.com

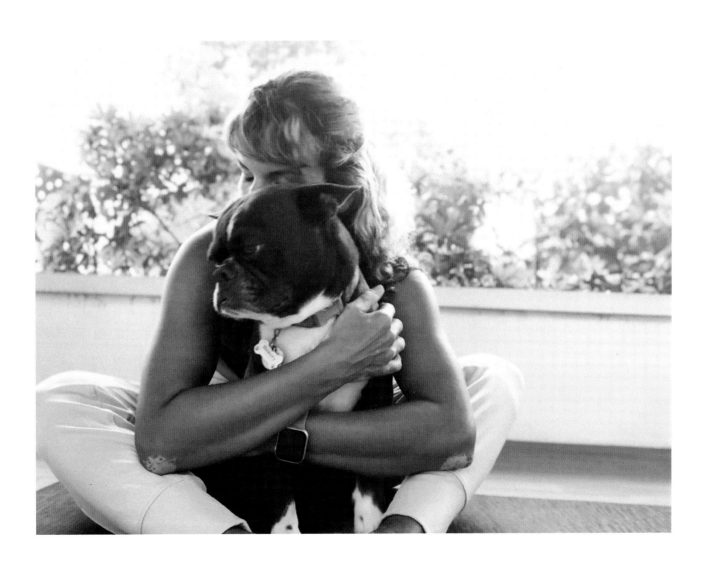